Autopsy - What Do We Learn from Corpses?

Edited by Kamil Hakan Dogan

Published in London, United Kingdom

Autopsy - What Do We Learn from Corpses?
http://dx.doi.org/10.5772/intechopen.95739
Edited by Kamil Hakan Dogan

Contributors
Anil Garg, Nisha Goyal, Massimo Montisci, Giovanni Cecchetto, Guido Viel, Carmen Cerda-Aguilar, William Aguilar-Navarro, Pooja Ahuja, Niha Ansari, Kamil Hakan Dogan

First published in London, United Kingdom, 2022 by IntechOpen
IntechOpen is the global imprint of INTECHOPEN LIMITED, registered in England and Wales, registration number: 11086078, 5 Princes Gate Court, London, SW7 2QJ, United Kingdom

British Library Cataloguing-in-Publication Data
A catalogue record for this book is available from the British Library

Additional hard and PDF copies can be obtained from orders@intechopen.com

Autopsy - What Do We Learn from Corpses?
Edited by Kamil Hakan Dogan
p. cm.
Print ISBN 978-1-80355-339-9
Online ISBN 978-1-80355-340-5
eBook (PDF) ISBN 978-1-80355-341-2

Meet the editor

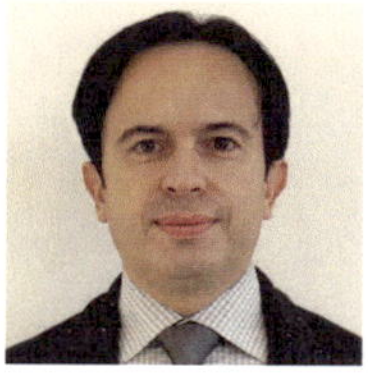

Kamil Hakan Dogan MD, Ph.D., is a full professor and chair in the Faculty of Medicine, Department of Forensic Medicine, Selcuk University, Turkey. Dr. Dogan received his MD from the Faculty of Medicine, Gazi University, Turkey in 2000. He received his Ph.D. in Biochemistry in 2012. He gives lectures on forensic medicine and medical ethics to medical students as well as students of the dentistry and law faculties. He is the editor of five books and *Bulletin of Legal Medicine* and a reviewer for several international journals. He has published more than 200 articles in refereed journals, chapters in textbooks, and abstracts in scientific meetings. His publications have been cited more than 1000 times.

Contents

Preface

The postmortem examination remains a benchmark in the study of human disease and is a vital tool for teaching anatomy to medical students. If the death is suspicious, a postmortem examination of the body is performed with the intent of determining the cause and manner of the death. Forensic medicine explores the legal aspects of medicine, and the medicolegal investigation of death is its most significant and crucial function. There is a keen interest among forensic medicine experts and the public in the advancements in forensic medicine. The nature of postmortem examinations is changing and the understanding of causes of death is evolving with the increase of knowledge and availability and use of various analyses including genetic testing. Postmortem examination practice is developing a more multidisciplinary approach to investigations, which are becoming more evidence-based.

Death scene investigation, postmortem examination, and autopsy are generally performed for the benefit of the living. A death investigation begins with body examination and evidence collection at the scene and proceeds through history, postmortem examination and autopsy, laboratory tests, and determining the cause and manner of death. Forensic pathology is the oldest branch of the forensic sciences, and today many branches of forensic sciences play a role in solving criminal death cases.

This book provides some basic information on postmortem examination and autopsy. It is useful for forensic pathologists, clinicians, attorneys, law enforcement officers, and medical students. I gratefully acknowledge the help and support of the authors from four continents who contributed to this book.

Dr. Kamil Hakan Dogan
Faculty of Medicine,
Department of Forensic Medicine,
Selcuk University,
Konya, Turkey

Chapter 1

Introductory Chapter: An Overview of the Autopsy Procedure

Kamil Hakan Dogan

1. Introduction

Forensic medicine is a branch of medicine that applies the principles and knowledge of the medical sciences to problems in the field of law [1]. It is the application of medical knowledge for the scientific investigation of facts and causal relationships, as well as the analysis and interpretation thereof in the service of the law in its broadest sense; moreover, it addresses all legal aspects of the practice of medicine during teaching, medical training, and specialist training. From a historical perspective, "forensic" or "medicolegal" medicine has grown as a scientific medical specialty primarily to assist police and legal authorities by providing expert appraisals in the fact-finding and adjudication process. The investigative and appraisal activities inherent to forensic medicine are required far beyond the purposes of criminal prosecution and thus make an important contribution in terms of legal certainty and a functioning rule of law. Forensic medicine is traditionally concerned foremost with the investigation of sudden and unexpected deaths. The focus here is on determining the mode of death on the basis of the established cause of death. In this context and besides unnatural deaths apparent at first glance, sudden natural deaths as well as a large group of unexplained deaths need to be considered [2].

The major duties of a medicolegal system in handling deaths falling under its jurisdiction are to determine the cause and manner of death, identify the deceased if unknown, determine the time of death and injury, collect evidence from the body that can be used to prove or disprove an individual's guilt or innocence, and confirm or deny the account of how the death occurred, document injuries, or lack of them, deduce how the injuries occurred, document any natural disease present, determine or exclude other contributory or causative factors to the death, and provide expert testimony if the case goes to trial [1].

2. The cause of death and the manner of death

The cause of death is the disease or injury, which sets in motion the physiologic train of events culminating in cerebral and cardiac electrical silence. The manner of death is a pseudojudicial classification of deaths dating back to Norman England, when the property of suicide victims was seized by the Crown. The four manners of death are natural, accident, suicide, and homicide [3]. The forensic determination of cause of death in natural deaths relates primarily to deaths involving, for example, suspicious circumstances in which a body is found or any other circumstances that may require the authorities to determine the cause of death. In such cases, the spectrum of diseases

IntechOpen

causally linked to (sudden) death is broad: myocardial infarct, myocarditis, coronary atherosclerosis with acute heart failure, ruptured aneurysm, pneumonia, meningitis, etc. Death is also often caused by relatively rare diseases, which, due to acute death and failure of the patient to seek medical advice, remained undiagnosed during the individual's lifetime [2]. In many cases, the cause and manner of death may be obvious. It is the documentation of the injuries or lack of them, as well as the interpretation of how they occurred and the determination or exclusion of other contributory or causative factors that are important [1].

3. The difference between forensic autopsy and medical autopsy

Autopsies have served numerous purposes for decades, including: determining underlying disease and cause of death in the individual case, expanding scientific knowledge (e.g., metastatic behavior of malignancies), assessing disease response to therapy, comparing autopsy findings with diagnostic findings, gaining insight into the evolution of new diseases (HIV infection, AIDS, SIRS, etc.), revealing and explaining hitherto unknown aspects of forensic criminological and insurance medicine, and in the education, training, and further training of medical students, medical assistants, and physicians in specialist medical training or other forms of further training [2]. An autopsy represents a postmortem surgical examination of a human body, but not all autopsies are equivalent. There are two basic types of autopsies: forensic or medicolegal autopsies and hospital or medical autopsies [4].

The forensic autopsy differs from the hospital or medical autopsy in its objectives and relevance. Besides determining the cause of death, the forensic pathologist must establish the manner of death (natural, accidental, suicidal, or homicidal), the identity of the deceased if unknown, and the time of death or injury. The forensic autopsy may also involve collection of evidence from the body, which can subsequently be used to either prove or disprove an individual's guilt, and confirm or deny his account of how the death occurred [1].

4. What should be considered when performing a forensic autopsy?

In the broadest sense, a forensic or medicolegal autopsy is any autopsy that generates an evidentiary document that forms a basis for opinions rendered in a criminal trial, deposition, wrongful death civil suit, medical malpractice civil suit, administrative hearing, or workmen's compensation hearing [3]. The forensic autopsy involves not only the actual examination of the body at the autopsy table, but the consideration of other aspects that the general pathologist does not believe to be part of the autopsy—the scene, clothing, and toxicology. The forensic autopsy begins at the scene. Pathologists should not perform a forensic autopsy unless they know the circumstances leading up to and surrounding the death. This is a very basic principle that is often violated [1]. Not examining a body at the scene has been considered a potential pitfall for the pathologist in a medicolegal death investigation. Scene visitation is not always necessary or possible for a pathologist conflicted by other duties. Death scene and witness information from different investigators (coroner, medical examiner or investigator, police, fire marshal, etc.) can be communicated to the pathologist by various means (diagrams, photographs, video, and digital images) prior to the autopsy [5].

What would one think of a physician who examined a patient without asking what the patient's symptoms or complaints were? As in all examinations of patients, one must have a medical history. In the case of the forensic pathologist, the "patient" is unable to render this history. Therefore, the history must be obtained by other investigators. This history should be known before the autopsy begins. The scene should be documented either with diagrams or photographs, preferably both. People should be interviewed, and a written report should be given to the pathologist prior to the autopsy. The body should be touched and moved as little as possible at the scene. In cases of violent death, paper bags should be secured about the victim's hands so that no trace evidence will be lost. Prior to transportation, the body should be either wrapped in a clean white sheet or placed in a clean body bag. Examination of the clothing is as much a part of the autopsy as examination of the wounds. The clothing must be examined for blood stains and trace evidence as well as to see if the wounds in the body correlate with the defects in the clothing [1].

5. Conclusions

Many medicolegal death investigations rely on information derived from autopsies. The success of an autopsy in answering questions (e.g., identification, injury causation) depends on a systematic approach by the pathologist. The "complete autopsy" is a series of necessary steps taken by the pathologist, who receives background information about the deceased, performs an external examination and internal dissection, and collects appropriate bodily samples for supplementary testing. The care exercised by the pathologist in this process is reflected in an accurate autopsy report, which addresses the most important question—the cause of death. The pathologist must be aware of potential pitfalls at every step of the postmortem investigation, any of which can pose a risk to the final resolution of a medicolegal investigation [5].

Author details

Kamil Hakan Dogan
Faculty of Medicine, Selcuk University, Konya, Turkey

*Address all correspondence to: drhakan2000@gmail.com

References

[1] Dimaio VJM, Molina DK. DiMaio's Forensic Pathology. 3rd ed. Boca Raton: CRC Press; 2021. DOI: 10.4324/9780429318764

[2] Dettmeyer RB, Verhoff MA, Schütz HF. Forensic Medicine: Fundamentals and Perspectives. Berlin: Springer-Verlag; 2014. DOI: 10.1007/978-3-642-38818-7

[3] Waters BL. Handbook of Autopsy Practice. 4th ed. Totowa: Humana Press; 2009. DOI: 10.1007/978-1-59745-127-7

[4] Prahlow J. Forensic Pathology for Police, Death Investigators, Attorneys, and Forensic Scientists. New York: Springer-Verlag; 2010. DOI: 10.1007/978-1-59745-404-9

[5] Shkrum MJ, Ramsay DA. Forensic Pathology of Trauma: Common Problems for the Pathologist. Totowa: Humana Press; 2007. DOI: 10.1007/978-1-59745-138-3

Chapter 2

External Examination of the Corpse

William Aguilar-Navarro and Carmen Cerda-Aguilar

Abstract

The autopsy and the external examination of the corpse become a decisive instance when resolving issues of various matters related to an individual. Its aim is not only to establish a diagnosis, but also to provide information about facts related to an illness or legal proceedings. The main tasks of this analysis are firstly to establish death and then to determine the cause and manner of death.

Keywords: external examination, corpse, cause, death

1. Introduction

The external examination of the corpse is a procedure that can provide information on the examination of the body when the identity is unknown, provides guidance on cause of death, unnatural, or unexplained manner of death, and determines conditions, for example, time of death [1].

The external examination of the body must be accurate and must be performed by trained people with many years of experience in the field, as sometimes medical work is combined with the forensic work.

During the external examination, definitive signs of death (temperature, lividity, rigor, or advanced postmortem changes) should be considered. In the procedure, all areas of the naked body should be analyzed and photographed, and all visual evidence and findings, such as scars, traumatic changes, tattoos, deformities, syringe marks, should be reported [2].

Unnatural deaths are those with external influence, due to physical aggression, accident, homicide, poisoning, suicide, and in those death, the external examination is very important, because it can provide information about the cause, with indicators on the body such as conjunctival hemorrhages, livor mortis color, signs of injury, among others [1].

For these reasons, the external examination of the corpse is of great importance, as it allows to:

- To provide the elements of identification.
- Plan the steps to be followed in an autopsy, for which it is necessary to determine the autopsy technique to obtain results according to the needs of the case.
- Document any pathological findings from the outset.

IntechOpen

- Support a medico-legal case if a full autopsy is not possible (which has happened due to health regulations in the context of the COVID-19 pandemic).
- Provide evidence in cases of allegations of lack of timely and adequate obstetric care.
- Document cases of neglected of elderly, disabled adults, and young children in the care of third parties.

2. External examination of the corpse

2.1 Identification elements

In addition to fingerprints, there are other elements accessible for external examination that can be valuable in determining or also confirming the identification of the deceased, such as dental features and tattoos [3]. In the case of dental features, age, sex, habits, cultural characteristics can be determined (**Figure 1**) in addition to the identification of the individual by comparison with dental records [4]. In the case of tattoos, it is important as a complement for identification (**Figure 2**), as it can provide information for relatives or a tour of tattoo shops which can narrow down the search field [5].

2.2 Autopsy step plan

Before performing an autopsy, it is ideal is to obtain as much information as possible, such as the place where the body or remains were discovered, the circumstances of death, the postmortem interval, the history of previous illnesses, and whether it was a witnessed death.

But if this is not possible, elements of external examination may be useful to:

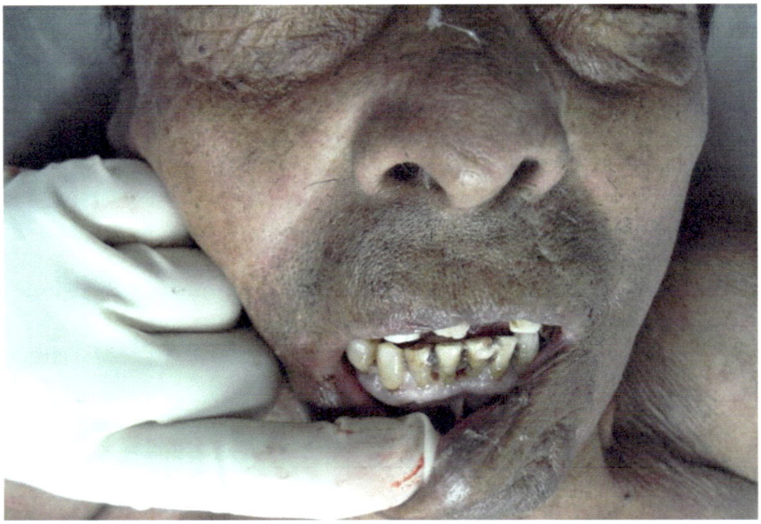

Figure 1.
Denture with missing pieces and poor care conditions.

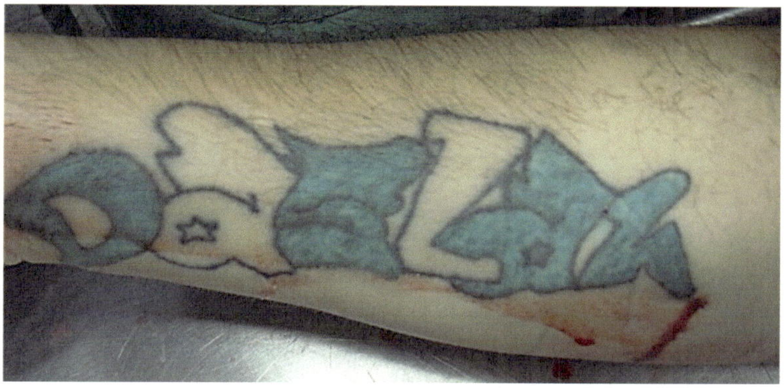

Figure 2.
Oversized and eye-catching tattoo.

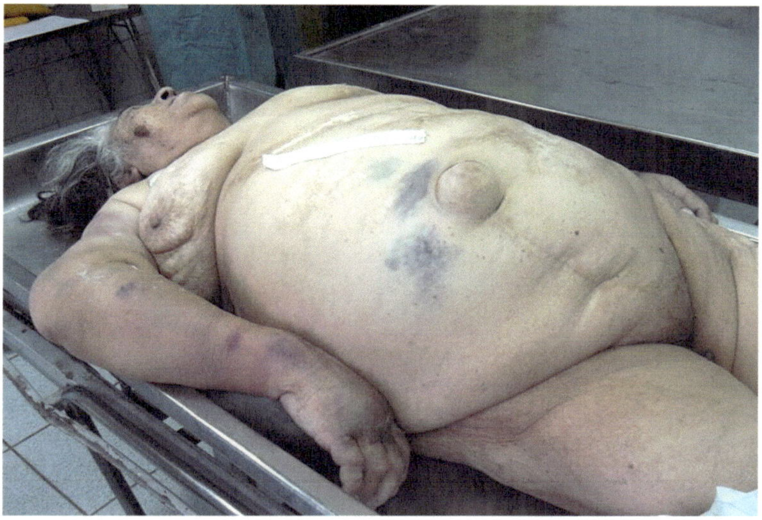

Figure 3.
Large umbilical hernia, with a median infra-umbilical laparotomy scar. The autopsy incision should be lateralised to visualize the underlying structures without interrupting them.

- Take extreme precautions in the use of personal protective equipment if infection is suspected.
- Establish where the incisions will be placed, so as not to compromise internal structures (**Figure 3**).
- Establish before starting the autopsy procedure, which complementary tests may be necessary, to have the appropriate containers (e.g., Petri dishes with culture media, fixatives for electron microscopy studies) or to establish coordination with other laboratories, in cases that require quickly processing.
- The existence of entry points for skin infection, such as pressure ulcers (bed sores), suggests that sepsis may be present (**Figure 4**). Staining for microorganisms such as Gram stain and Lactophenol Blue needs to be considered [6, 7].

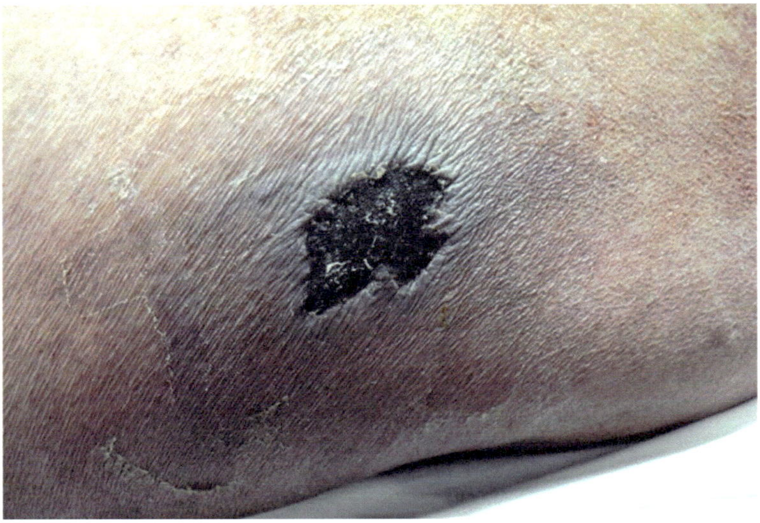

Figure 4.
Decubitus ulcer (pressure or bed sores). It is a starting point for skin sepsis.

2.3 Documenting any pathological findings from the outset

Many external signs in the ocular conjunctiva, mucosa of the lips, teeth, ears, or skin, among others, may suggest the underlying disease, or be a key in differential diagnoses.

Internal examination findings only have an impact on the clinicopathological picture, causing or contributed to death.

Alterations in skin color, focal such as petechiae or ecchymosis (**Figures 5** and **6**) or diffuse such as jaundice, the presence of edema (**Figure 7**), suggest from external

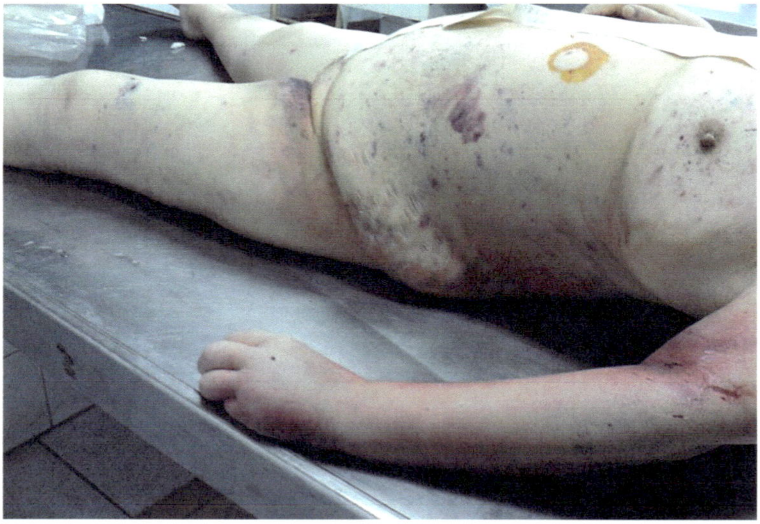

Figure 5.
Petechiae on the chest and left flank. Thrombocytopenic purpura.

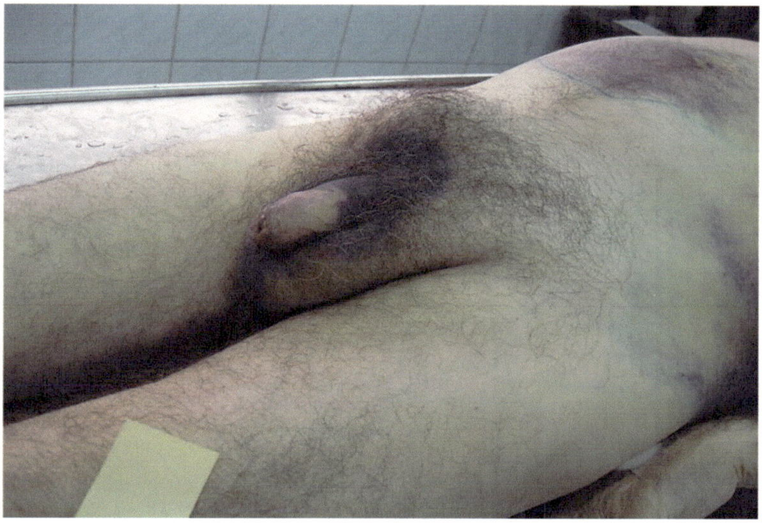

Figure 6.
Extensive ecchymoses on the abdomen, pubic and genital region. Coagulopathy by anticoagulants.

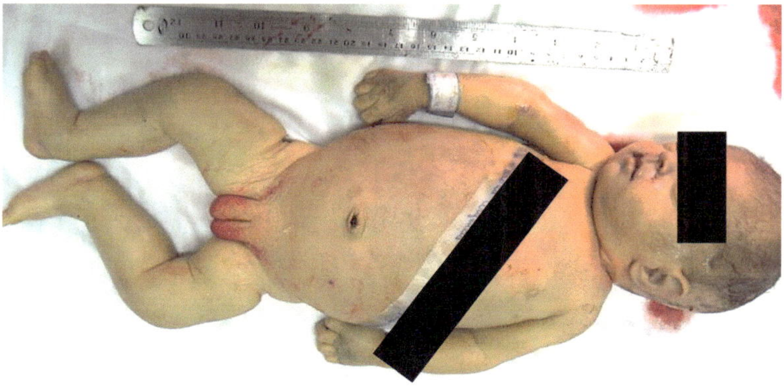

Figure 7.
Jaundice and generalized edema. Stillborn with Rh incompatibility and isoimmunization.

examination of the body that it will be necessary to study certain organs and systems, both macroscopically and through complementary tests, like imaging, histopathology, forensic histopathology, or molecular biology.

An example of this is how histology and forensic histopathology can be of great use in the diagnosis of skin alterations, which can give us an understanding of lesions or postmortem changes in the structure of the skin [8].

In congestive heart failure and myocardial infarction, vasodilation and congestion are observed, especially in the mucous membranes and conjunctivae, due to their transparency (**Figure 8**).

When pallor is severe, massive hemorrhage must be presumed. Occasionally, the source of bleeding is an external injury, as well as the gastrointestinal or respiratory tract (**Figure 9**).

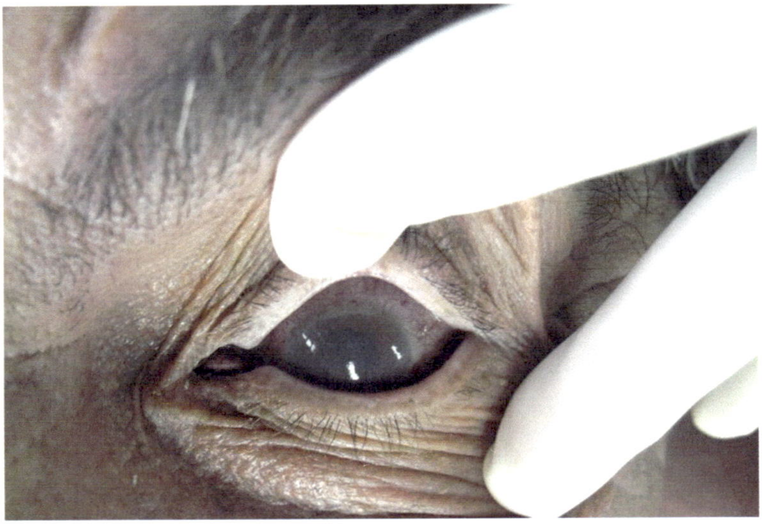

Figure 8.
Conjunctival congestion. Acute myocardial infarction.

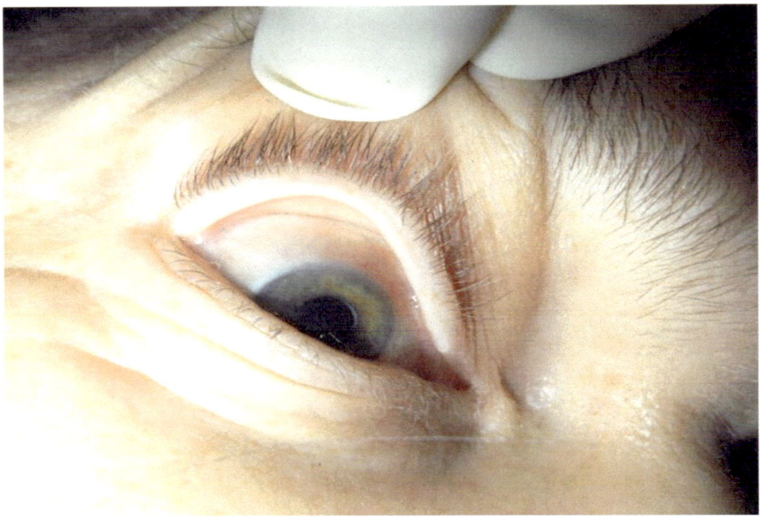

Figure 9.
Conjunctival pallor. Cutting wound.

2.4 Support a medico-legal case if a full autopsy is not possible

In response to the COVID-19 pandemic, many countries have adapted their regulations on the examination of the deceased, reducing and eventually banning clinical autopsies [9, 10].

Forensic services, for their part, have restricted forensic autopsies, subjecting them to autopsy in case of a negative PCR for COVID-19, or even leaving the decision to prosecutors who do not usually handle technical criteria.

Therefore, forensic autopsies of potential cases and especially of confirmed cases, especially those without signs of violence, should be kept to a minimum and performed only when necessary, and internal examination of the body should be carried out only when necessary [11].

As it is necessary to have a cause of death to initiate a legal process and bring the case to justice, we can use the alternatives at our disposal to support the decision whether to do an autopsy and take certain samples.

In cases of sudden death, there is usually no history, so an autopsy and other complementary tests will be necessary, such as histopathology.

Deaths caused by trauma, asphyxia, and poisoning are classified as violent. A thorough external examination may be sufficient to document a case of violent death, for example:

- In cases of traumatic death, where the offending element is often external to the body, it is essential to document the type, size, location, and relationship between external injuries. And non-invasive imaging tests may be useful.

- If the presence of cyanosis suggests asphyxia, manual asphyxia and all lessons accompanied by constriction of the neck should be documented by photographs of the respective groove, fingerprints, nail stigmata, lividity studies, and lividity arrangement in cases of incomplete suspension.

- Only if there are doubts about submersion asphyxia, it is necessary to prove the presence of a foreign body in the airway, which may require an internal examination.

- In the case of poisoning, it should be borne in mind that for analysis and demonstration, it is necessary to isolate the toxic substance from the tissues or fluids of the corpse, for which it is essential to take a good sample. Although toxic substances produce what is called "asphyxia," visible changes on external examination may be of value: Lividity of colors, other purplish spots, miosis, increased facial congestion are characteristic of some poisonings.

In cases of gunshot wounds, it is very important to determine the distance of the shot, the angle of the shot, the position in which the victim was when the projectile hit, and the entry and exit orifices (**Figures 10** and **11**).

In cases of asphyxia due to aspiration of gastric contents, in addition to cyanosis, the cause of death may be evident on external examination (**Figures 12** and **13**).

2.5 Evidence in cases of allegations of lack of obstetric care

Autopsy of newborns can provide information to physicians and families about the cause of death and the accuracy of the antemortem clinical diagnosis [12].

Some women have given birth to a newborn. These deaths are attributed to excessive delay in obstetric care and lack of control of the fetoplacental unit. It is essential to record the external features of the stillbirth body to establish the approximate date of death in utero and the gestational age [13, 14].

Routine external examination includes body measurements (at least: body weight, crown-rump length, crown-heel length, foot length, occipitofrontal circumference).

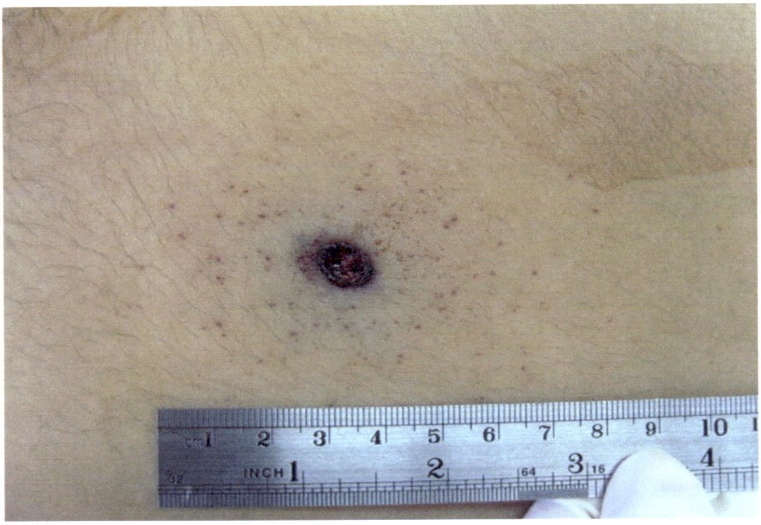

Figure 10.
Close-range shot, with concentric equimotic-erosive halo and gunshot residue encrustation on its periphery.

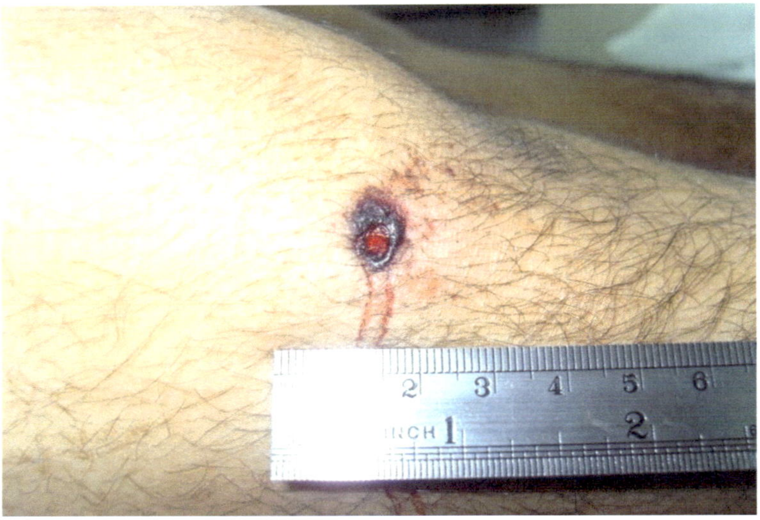

Figure 11.
Long distance shot, no residue, with eccentric equimotic-erosive halo.

Detailed external examination, including nutritional status/soft tissue and muscle volume; the presence of edema (localized/generalized), pallor, meconium staining, jaundice or the presence of trauma, location of thoracic drains and vascular cannulae, and other iatrogenic lesions (**Figures 14** and **15**) [15].

The report should include a description of the external morphology specifically mentioning fontanelles, eyes, ears, nose, choanal patency, palatal fusion, spine, extremities, fingers, palmar creases, external genitalia, anal patency, umbilical cord [15]. It is used to diagnose, why some fetuses die in the prenatal period due incompatible life malformations (**Figures 16–18**) [16].

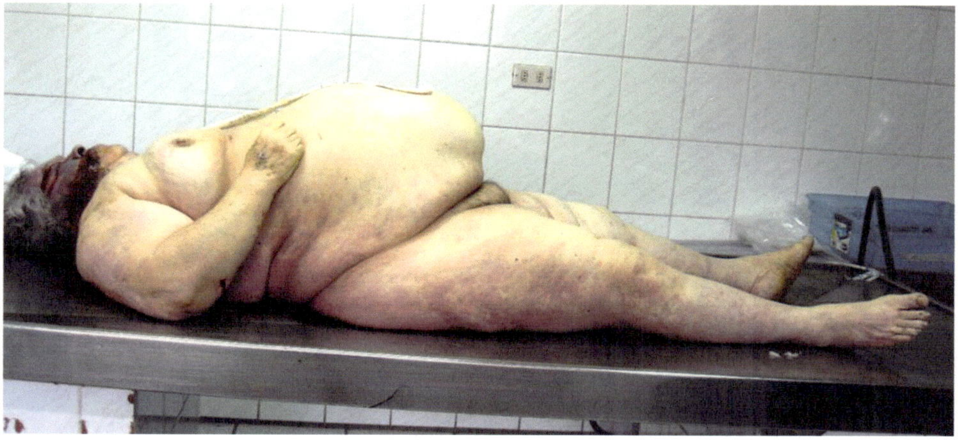

Figure 12.
Patient found dead at home. Morbid obesity with complicated umbilical hernia, and intestinal volvulus.

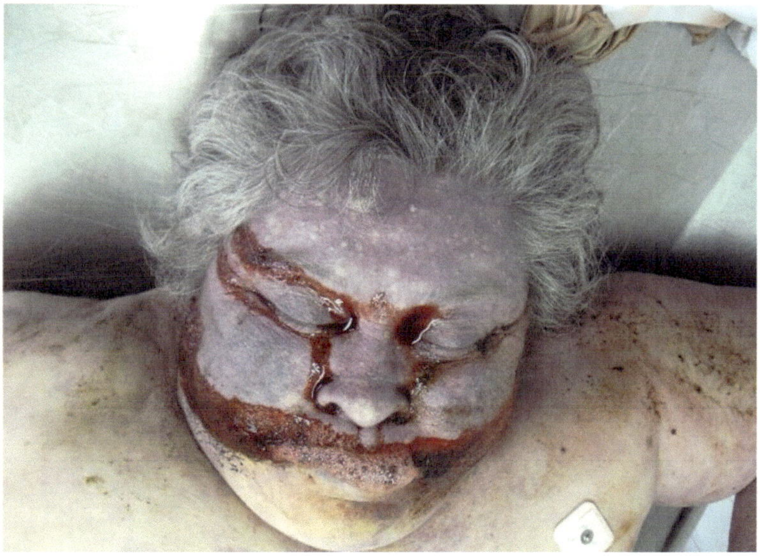

Figure 13.
The same patient with severe cyanosis. Foamy hemorrhagic coming out of the mouth and nose.

Examination of the ovarian adnexa may also clarify the causes of death, such as large retroplacental clots (premature detachment of the placenta), opaque ovarian membranes (indicating ovarian infection), or true knots in the umbilical cord (**Figure 19**) [17, 18].

2.6 Document cases of neglected of elderly, disabled adults, and young children in the care of third parties

Malnutrition, soiling, bed sores and colonization by insects on living persons [19, 20] are located on the conjunctivae, ulcers, genitalia, or other wounds (**Figure 20**).

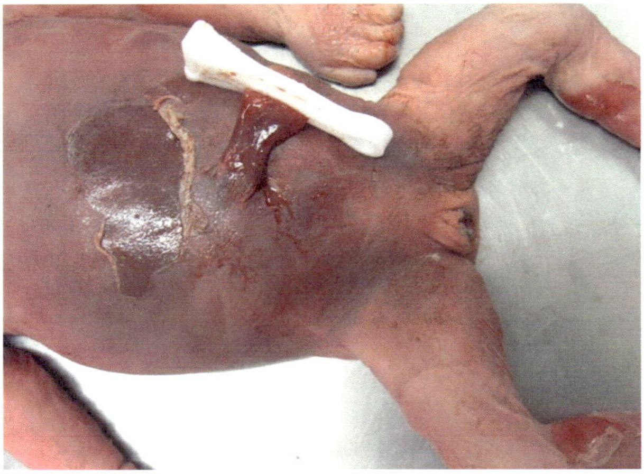

Figure 14.
Premature stillbirth. With skin. Sloughing.

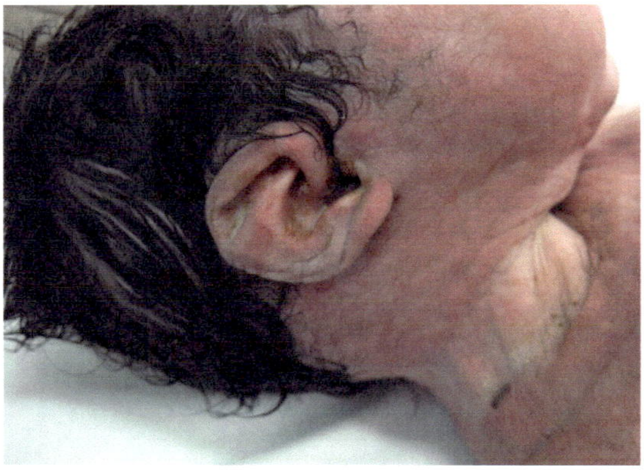

Figure 15.
Term newborn. Fully developed pinna.

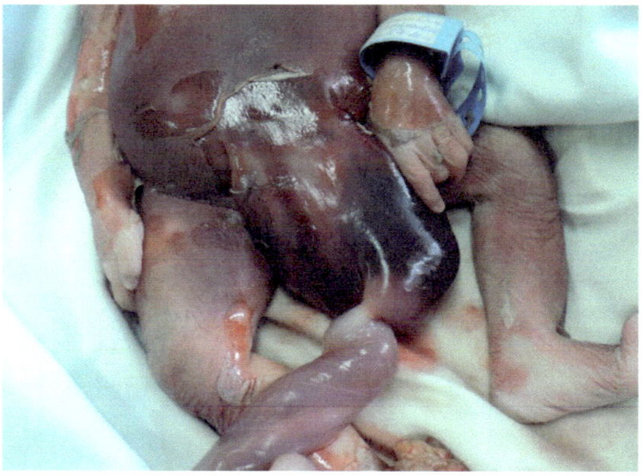

Figure 16.
Premature and macerated fetus with large omphalocele.

These are the elements that in a judicial process that allow proving the crime of abandonment or neglect of vulnerable people by their relatives or caregivers. An example of poor care is best illustrated by the diagnosis of marasmus and cachexia. These diseases were frequently diagnosed. They were only rarely cited as a cause of death [21].

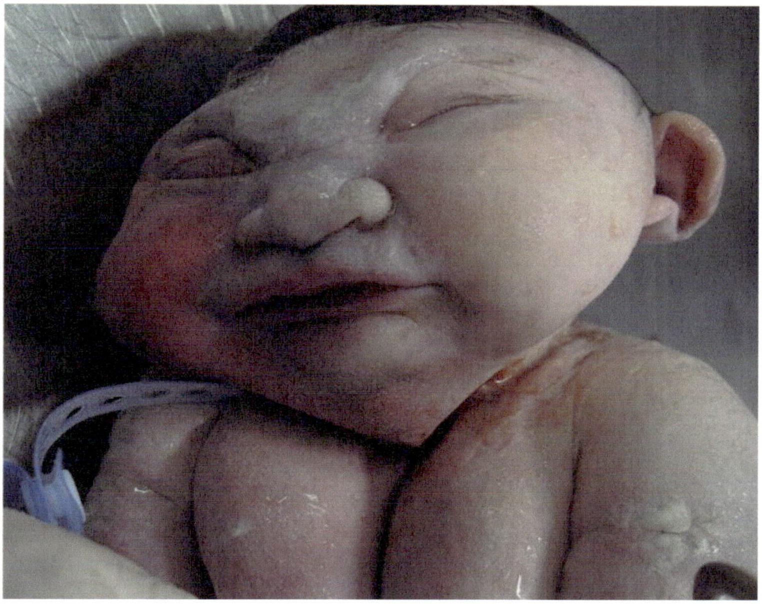

Figure 17.
Term newborn, with multiple head and body malformations.

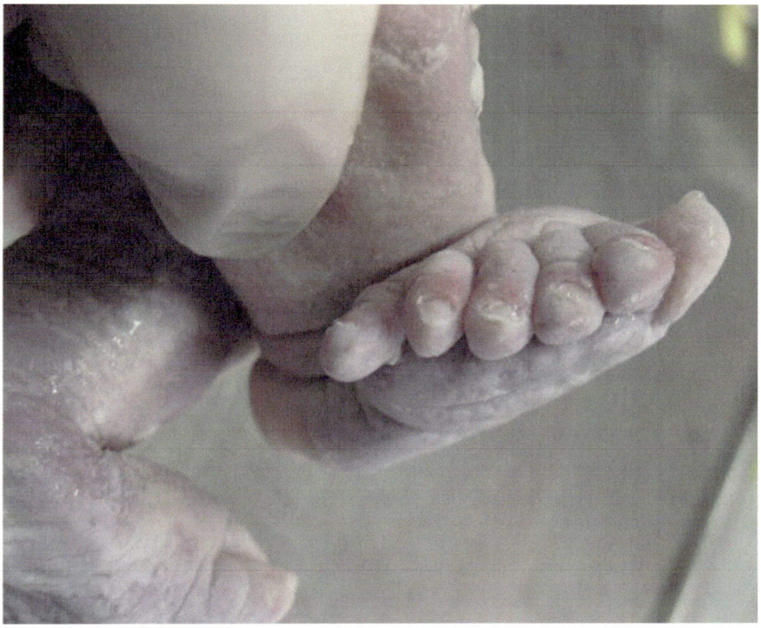

Figure 18.
Term newborn, with foot malformations.

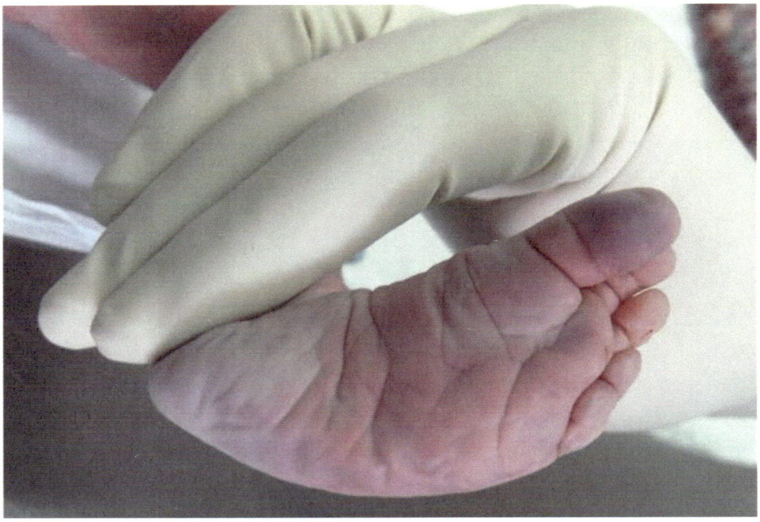

Figure 19.
Malformation of the foot secondary to oligohydramnios. This condition is associated with polycystic kidney or renal agenesis.

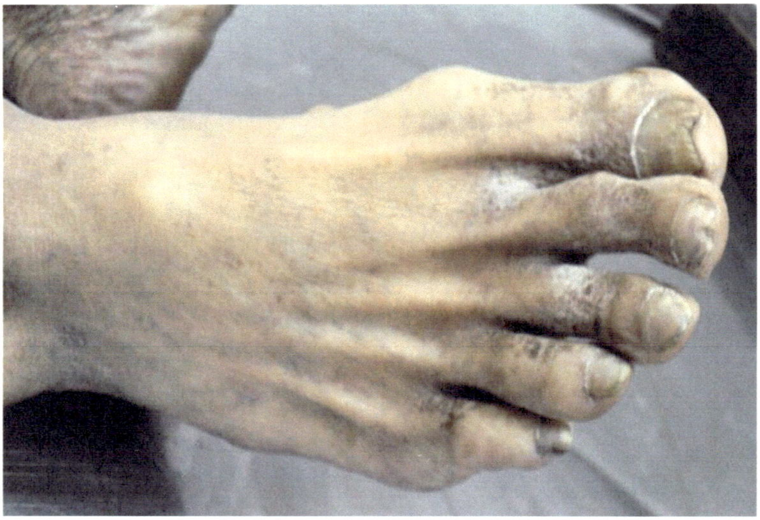

Figure 20.
Elderly adult male, living in a nursing home. Malnutrition, dirt, and dermatophytosis.

3. Conclusions

Despite the evolution of imaging techniques, the postmortem examination has maintained a key role in the clinical and forensic analysis. To obtain reliable information on the types of death and to allow a better understanding of the phenomenon, it is useful to study the results of clinical and forensic autopsies that start with the external examination of the corpse.

The search for and documentation of seemingly small details in the external examination of corpses help to resolve difficult situations surrounding medico-legal deaths, such as the identification of undocumented victims, the cause and manner of death, the postmortem interval, differential diagnoses of the cause of death, or the regulation of not performing complete autopsies during health crises.

Author details

William Aguilar-Navarro* and Carmen Cerda-Aguilar
University of Chile, Santiago, Chile

*Address all correspondence to: waguilar@uchile.cl

References

[1] Madea B. The postmortem external examination. Deutsches Ärzteblatt International. 2021;**107**(33):575-588. DOI: 10.3238/arztebl.2010.0575

[2] Arslan M. Handbook of Forensic Autopsy: Basic Algorithms and Technique. Independently published; 2021. p. 278. ISBN-13: 979-8759840022

[3] Marín L, Moreno F. Odontología Forense. Identificación odontológica de cadáveres quemados. Reporte de dos casos. Revista Estomatología; 2004;**12**(2):57-70

[4] Nambiar P. Identification from dental characteristics. The Medical Journal of Malaysia. 1995;**49**:406-408

[5] Birngruber CG, Martinez Peña EG, Corrales Blanco L, et al. The use of tattoos to identify unknown bodies. Rechtsmedizin. 2020;**30**:219-224. DOI: 10.1007/s00194-020-00396-y

[6] López-Jácome LE, Hernández-Durán M, Colín-Castro CA, Ortega-Peña S, et al. Las tinciones básicas en el laboratorio de microbiología. Investigación en Discapacidad. 2014;**3**(1)

[7] Araiza J, Hernández M. Procedimientos y técnicas de diagnóstico. In: Bonifaz Trujillo J, editor. Micología médica básica 5 ed. Ciudad de México: McGraw Hill Interamericana Editores. 2015. Available from: https://accessmedicina.mhmedical.com/content.aspx?bookid=1529&sectionid=98870458

[8] Wei W, Michu Q, Wenjuan D, et al. Histological changes in human skin 32 days after death and the potential forensic significance. Scientific Reports. 2020;**10**:18753. DOI: 10.1038/s41598-020-76040-2

[9] Organismo de Investigación Judicial. Lineamientos generales para el manejo de los cadáveres que requieren autopsia médico legal en los casos en investigación, probables o confirmados de COVID-19 en el Marco de la alerta sanitaria por coronavirus (COVID-19). República de Costa Rica. Poder Judicial; 2020;**1**:1-10

[10] Henwood AF. Coronavirus disinfection in histopathology. Journal of Histotechnology. 2020;**43**:102-104. DOI: 10.1080/01478885.2020.1734718

[11] González-Fernández J, Ibáñez-Bernáldez M, Martínez-Tejedor JA, Alama-Carrizo S, Sánchez-Ugena F, Montero-Juanes JM. Gestión de los cadáveres durante la pandemia por COVID-19 en España. Revista Española de Medicina Legal. 2020;**46**:109-118. DOI: 10.1016/j.reml.2020.05.001

[12] de Sévaux JLH, Nikkels PGJ, Lequin MH, Groenendaal F. The value of autopsy in neonates in the 21st century. Neonatology. 2019;115:89-93. DOI: 10.1159/000493003

[13] Moore IE. Macerated stillbirth. In: Keeling JW, Khong TY, editors. Fetal and Neonatal Pathology. London: Springer; 2007. DOI: 10.1007/978-1-84628-743-5_10

[14] Gold KJ, Abdul-Mumin AR, Boggs ME, Opare-Addo HS, Lieberman RW. Assessment of "fresh" versus "macerated" as accurate markers of time since intrauterine fetal demise in low-income countries. International Journal of Gynecology & Obstetrics. 2014;**125**:223-227

[15] Osborn M. Guidelines on Autopsy Practice: Neonatal Death. London: The Royal College of Pathologists; 2019

[16] International Journal of Gynaecology and Obstetrics: The Official Organ of the International Federation of Gynaecology and Obstetrics. 2014;**125**:223-227. DOI: 10.1016/j. ijgo.2013.12.006

[17] Aspillaga C, Las Heras J, Kakarieka E, Avila R, Henríquez C. Anomalías del cordón umbilical y su asociación con malformaciones fetales [anomalies of the umbilical cord and its association with fetal malformations]. Revista Chilena de Obstetricia y Ginecología. 1991;**56**(1): 27-34 Spanish

[18] Hammad IA et al. Umbilical cord abnormalities and stillbirth. Obstetrics and Gynecology. 2020;**135**(3):644-652. DOI: 10.1097/AOG.0000000000003676

[19] Vanin S et al. A case of insect colonization before the death. Journal of Forensic Sciences. 2017;**62**:1665-1667. DOI: 10.1111/1556-4029.13481

[20] Kotzé Z et al. The forensic entomology case report—A global perspective. Insects. 2021;**12**:283. DOI: 10.3390/insects12040283

[21] Klima M et al. Causes of death in geriatric patients: A cross-cultural study. Journal of Gerontology. 1997;**4**:247-253

Chapter 3

Post-Mortem Assessment and Evolutionary Role of the Autopsy

Massimo Montisci, Giovanni Cecchetto and Guido Viel

Abstract

The Chapter is dedicated to the evolutionary role of autopsy, reporting the historical profiles, the state of the art, and prospects for future development of the main related techniques and methods of the ancillary disciplines (like Radiology), involved in historic synergy in the post-mortem assessment, together with the mother discipline Forensic Pathology. A task sustainable through the utilization of the so-called advanced molecular autopsy, a convergence of different skills jointly makes use of the high dimensionality of data generated by new technologies requiring a data mining approach governed by improved bioinformatics and computational biology tools. The evolution of the scientific research and the increased accuracy of the various disciplines will be able to weigh the value of evidence, placed at the disposal of the justice system as truth and proof.

Keywords: medicolegal autopsy, forensic autopsy, post-mortem assessment, forensic pathology, radiology, and imaging

1. Introduction

The autopsy is the dissection of the dead body to determine the cause of death or the nature of the disease [1].

In particular, the anatomical or anatomical-pathological autopsies aims to study the human morphology and to improve the knowledge among students of medicine [2]. The forensic autopsies are requested by police, prosecutor, coroner, or judge, to solve specific problems, not only the cause of death (natural or traumatic), but also the manner of death (homicide, suicide, accidental), the time of death and sometime the identity of the deceased [3].

Unfortunately, in the past half century the rate of autopsies conducted throughout much of the world declined [2]. In the past, usually the pathologist revealed the diseased anatomy of patients. Such activity confirmed or disproved diagnoses, permitted assessment of the effects and appropriateness of treatment, and illustrated the relentless advance of disease.

The experience could be humbling or reassuring, but it was always a deterrent to medical hubris. Autopsies were a form of audit for the whole medical team, including internists, surgeons, and radiologists. With a reduced emphasis on autopsies, the skills required for performing these procedures and reliably interpreting associated histopathology risk being eroded, and a time-honored form of quality control is being lost [4].

Globally, the reasons for decreased reliance on autopsies are diverse. They include an emphasis on reducing health care and educational costs; altered working patterns for pathologists, who are spending more time engaged in surgical pathology; cultural aversion to interfering with cadavers; a belief that advances in imaging and other diagnostic and teaching methods have rendered autopsies obsolete except for medicolegal purposes; and concern among practitioners about litigation if errors are identified during post-mortem examination [5].

Studies have repeatedly demonstrated that rates of identification of diagnostic errors or unrecognized diagnoses have not decreased over time; an oft-cited estimate is that such mistakes are revealed in about 30% of autopsies. Various approaches representing less invasive and more limited investigations into causes of death have been explored, but we generally rely less at present on examining cadavers altogether. Estimates of overall and cause specific mortality are mostly derived from information collected while people are living. But there is much we can learn from the dead, for both clinical and public health purposes [4].

Some epidemiological studies showed in different countries a decline in autopsies for diagnostic purposes in favor of those of a judicial and, even, didactic nature [3].

It is therefore difficult to recognize autopsies conducted solely for medicolegal purposes, especially as the documentation on this subject is often dispersed in works, including those of a non-medical nature, that are difficult to uncover [6].

2. Autopsy techniques

The modern autopsy techniques were developed in the 19th century in Germany, when the observation of single organs was accompanied by removal of organs in four blocks: 1) neck, lungs, heart, and thoracic aorta; 2) liver, spleen, stomach, duodenum and pancreatic gland; 3) intestine and 4) kidneys, adrenals, the abdominal part of the aorta and pelvic organs. Such a "new" technique permitted the investigation of injuries in anatomical relation to the surrounding organs and structures [6]. Today, this method is usually applied and sometime adapted to the requirements of every single case for injury patterns, for example in case of neck trauma, traffic accident, SIDS [7, 8], death of pregnant women [9], death due to air embolism [10], sexual homicide [11] and medical malpractice [12].

Each autopsy should be preceded by an examination at the scene of death and followed, sometimes, by different types of radiological examinations (X-ray, CT, and MRI), to then perform a thorough external examination of the corpse with a complete internal examination, by opening all three body cavities [13].

Indeed, to contribute as much as possible to the prosecution of the guilty and the defense of the innocent, the forensic autopsy should be performed in a completely way (*"the only thing worse than no autopsy is a partial autopsy"*). In fact, an incomplete autopsy may require a subsequent exhumation of the body, because what may seem initially not important could be it for the resolution of the case [3].

An autopsy well performed require different measurements: body weight and length, chest circumference, weights of various organs to describe health state and in children cases the development. Regarding the "report", the first part must describe all the findings (normal or pathological) of the external and internal examination. The second part contains an initial assessment of the results. Additional investigations (eg radiological examinations, which as X-ray, CT and MRI;

chemico-toxicological or microbiological exams), which are deemed necessary for answering questions, must be listed.

Furthermore, should be sampled and stored during autopsy tissue specimens for histological and immunohistochemical exams, sometimes whole organs (e.g., brain, heart, lungs), wounds, body fluids and tissue specimens for toxicology, genetics, and microbiology. All of these must be stored under special conditions, at different temperatures and for varying periods, guaranteeing an adequate chain of custody.

3. Microscopic techniques

microscopic examination is necessary in all cases in which gross examination leads to conflicting results.

Stainings of interest for forensic purposes are: hematoxylin–eosin (HE) for hemorrhages, Prussian blue reaction and Quincke stain for hemosiderin; Hematoxylin-Orange, Weigert stain for fibrin for the thrombosis; Sudan III for fat embolism; Hematoxylin-Orange for inflammatory cells (leucocytes), carmine or Gentian violet for mast cells, Heidenhain iron hematoxylin stain and eosin for fibroblasts.

Concerning forensic histopathology, several experimental studies tried to find new stainings for the identification of metallization on skin electric marks [14], for the study of gunshot entrance wound and gunshot residues (i.e., Giemsa) [15], for the determination of glycogen in cardiac tissue (PAS - periodic acid Schiff).

The cerebral injuries or chronology of lesions were particularly studied with experimental enzymatic studies [16, 17].

In the last few years, the scanner electron microscopy (SEM) has opened new fields of research regarding the heart [18], the detection of gunshot residue [19] or the electric and thermal injuries [20]. Furthermore, transmission electron microscopy (TEM) was able to demonstrate the hemorrhages and of oedema in asphyxia deaths [21], and silicon in lung silicon embolism. The Laser scanning confocal microscope permitted the simultaneous observation of more fluorochromes and multidimensional analysis (2D, 3D and 4D) of the images, allowing to evaluate the activation stage of the cell and the detection of metals in tissues [22].

The environmental scanning electron microscopy has also permitted the analysis of materials or tissues without specimen preparation, to characterize saw or stab marks on bones [23] or detect diatoms in cases of drowning [24], in forensic cases of intoxications [25] or for the estimation of firing distance in gunshot-related deaths [26].

The immunohistochemistry (IHC) is mainly used in the analysis of the vitality and chronology of skin lesions or burned bodies, the chronology of cerebral hypoxia and myocardial ischemia and the diagnosis and duration of asphyxia, hypothermia, or hyperthermia [27].

The double-color immunofluorescence analysis combined with confocal microscopy is used for assessing the chronology of lesions and the cause of death in asphyxia cases [28].

In situ hybridization (ISH) is used in the identification of gender or in the search for viral DNA, for the study of the cases of diagnosis of SIDS [29].

Regarding histology, in the past it was recommended *"sections of normal and any abnormal areas of each organ for microscopic examination"* [30]; more recently all autopsies must performed a sampling of *"specimens from the main organs for histology*" [13], because the histology is fundamental for identifying and dating natural or traumatic disease, deaths related to acute or chronic exposure to xenobiotics [31], for reconstructing accidental or criminal dynamics [32] even in cases of medical malpractice [33].

4. Forensic radiology

Forensic Radiology have gained increasing importance in the field of Legal Medicine, but each method has its own advantages and limitations, that depend on the method used, the experience of the "legal radiologist". These kinds of exams were used to estimate the age and height of the victims, mainly for identification purposes [34].

4.1 Virtual autopsy

In 2000 the most famous project (the Virtopsy project) [35] opened the collaboration of the Legal Medicine with the Radiology in new systematic research combining both specialties in this field with the use of different basic techniques (conventional X-rays, CT, MRI) and complementary methods, like imaging-guided sampling, post-mortem angiography, and ultrasound, used to locate blood vessels for cannulation [36].

4.1.1 Conventional X-ray

It is the oldest technique of forensic imaging and has almost been eclipsed by the CT in modern imaging.

4.1.2 Computed tomography

The post-mortem CT (PMCT) is used to the reconstruction of two- and three-dimensional images, especially in examining the skeletal system. This method represents an excellent screening tool and adjunct to the conventional autopsy for: the high special resolution; rapid examination times (in only a few minutes permits the scanning of a whole body); easy handling of the CT unit; the possibility to detect any foreign material (projectiles and/or surgical material); the investigation and identification of victims (age and gender) of mass catastrophes [37]. The simple and clear images present accessible information to judges, police officers, and other individuals operating in the field of legal medicine [38].

However, the low contrast for organ visualization and the limited sensitivity for the detection of organ findings are the major downsides of the method, making it suitable for examining cases of traumatic death, such as firearm cases [39], but not natural death [40].

4.1.3 Magnetic resonance

MRI has the potential to overcome the limitations of PCMT, but it is only rarely used in forensic imaging because is a complex technology requiring specific training and high maintenance costs. The high soft-tissue resolution makes MRI a perfect tool for detecting natural causes of death (e.g., in the heart) and for examining traumatic soft-tissue injuries (e.g., in the brain).

4.1.4 Imaging-guided biopsies

These complements increase the sensibility of the radiological exam: imaging-guided biopsies or liquid aspiration, different matrices, organ tissue or body fluids can be obtained in a minimally invasive way, combining PMCT with histological, toxicological, or micro-biological investigations (e.g. collection and analysis of gas composition, distinguishing gas due to post-mortem decomposition from vital gas embolism or from other origins).

4.1.5 Angiography (PMA)

It is a promising method, that use an injection of contrast agent into the vascular system [41], selective (e.g., coronary arteries) or in a whole-body. PMA in combination with PMCT also leads to an increase of contrast in the soft tissue, allowing the detection of pathological findings. The most widespread technique is the multi-phase PMCT angiography (MPMCTA), that consists in the performance of a CT scan and after an injection of contrast agent (Angiofil®) with a perfusion device (Virtangio®). In this way the sensitivity of PMCT for detecting pathological findings in forensic cases can be increased from 65 to ~81%, very similar to a conventional autopsy, with important advantages in cases of sudden cardiac death (because it allows the detailed investigation of coronary arteries), fatal hemorrhage (because it permits the finding of even the smallest sources of bleeding), stab and gunshot trauma, and suspected medical error. Extra-vascular local application of contrast agent has been used to demonstrate the capacity to reconstruct stab directions and estimate the depth of the inflicted wounds [42].

4.1.6 Conclusion

In conclusion, for the detection of foreign bodies, PMCT or conventional X-ray techniques are most suitable and permit: rapid detection even in putrefied, carbonized, or otherwise highly damaged bodies; guidance for sampling the foreign bodies (e.g., projectiles); investigation of traumatic death, providing an information concerning the biomechanical origins of fractures for forensic reconstruction of the case. In cases of fatal hemorrhage, due to a sharp or gunshot trauma or suspected medical error, PMCT should be extended by adding whole-body PMCTA, that permits the discovery of the source of bleeding and the visualization of the trajectories of knives, needles, and projectiles. In cases of natural deaths, like sudden cardiac death, the methods of choice are MPMCTA, which permits a detailed investigation of stenosis or other lesions of the coronary arteries, and MRI, which shows the myocardium and eventual lesions within it.

4.2 Micro-radiology and future

Micro-radiology may prove to be the bridge that connects histopathology and diagnostic imaging as subspecialty of its own [43] and its use in forensic sciences is growing. The leading application is the structural study of calcified tissues, permitting the measurement and calculation of mineral density, volume, and surface, allowed to identify lesions, fractures, or dislocations of bones or calcified tissues [44]. In this way, this technique could inform on the morphology of tool marks on bone, on vitality and timing of fractures, and on age identification.

Micro-CT and micro-MRI can also help to identification of fire victims and to estimate the age at death and the cremation temperature of burned human remains.

This technique can perform a tri-dimensional spatial distribution of gunshot residue particles, also in wounds covered by textiles or altered by putrefaction, fire, or water, for the diagnosis between entrance and exit lesions and for the estimation of the firing distance.

Micro-MRI imaging can allow the estimation of the neuronal loss related to age, cranial trauma, or degenerative diseases.

5. Specific autopsy procedures

In 2015 the European Council of Legal Medicine (ECLM) published a checklist to identify qualified forensic experts who perform professional services of a high-quality standard, successfully undergoing official accreditation/certification [45, 46].

The ECLM document helps to standardize the medico-legal examination about the determination of the manner and cause of death. In particular, the document provides that the specialists should have a good experience in Legal Medicine, be independent of the police or the prosecuting authorities, and should be in possession of all the necessary equipment to provide high quality reports. The document includes general aspects (administrative space, quality assurance, statistical reports) and specific aspects (scene investigation, external examination, performance of an autopsy, radiological, histological, toxicological exams). accreditation can be request by any institution to the president of the ECLM who then nominates two inspectors to check it. The standards reported in this document [45], which take up the previous recommendations of the Council of Europe [13], are those necessary to qualify the activity of a forensic pathology service.

6. Post-mortem interval (PMI)

The Post-Mortem interval (PMI) is one of the most important items in forensic investigation, above all in case of homicide o traumatic deaths.

We can identify two different objectives of PMI at the scene of violent death (e.g., homicide):

1. to give a preliminary opinion of the time of an assault.

2. To check whether PMI is consistent or inconsistent with the alibi of a suspect.

For estimating the PMI, different sources are used:

1. information from the environment in the vicinity of the body (e.g, date, and hour in a watch).

2. Anamnestic factors concerning the deceased's habits (e.g., work, activities).

3. Post-mortem changes.

DOI: http://dx.doi.org/10.5772/intechopen.103885

All sources of information on PMI always should be kept in mind.

In forensic medicine much research has been carried out on post-mortem changes. The progression of all post-mortem changes is influenced by many internal or external factors, mainly the ambient temperature. The longer the post-mortem interval, the less accurate is the estimation of the time since death based on post-mortem changes.

Various methods are proposed for estimating the PMI, in particular [47]:

1. physical processes, like body cooling and hypostasis.

2. Physicochemical processes, like rigor mortis.

3. Concentration changes of metabolites or substrates.

4. Autolysis with increase or decrease of analytes in various body fluids.

5. Putrefaction due to bacterial processes.

Furthermore, the methods for estimating the PMI are not only different but also have widely varying scientific value in terms of the underlying scientific background, the mode of investigation and the validation of the method.

The chemical and biochemical analysis after death of bodily fluids (and among these Vitreous Humor) is an important approach to assess the PMI.

Vitreous Humor (VH) is a chemically complex aqueous solution of carbohydrates, proteins, electrolytes, and other small molecules present in living organisms; this biofluid is useful tool for its isolated environment, preserved from bacterial contamination, decomposition, autolysis, and metabolic reactions. VH has been used as a biofluid for forensic purposes in different studies. A recent review [48] evaluated the chemical and biochemical advances with particular importance on the endogenous compounds present at the time of death and their modification over time, which are valuable for the PMI prediction and to also identify, sometime, the cause of death. This review confirms that the VH analysis, especially the dosage of its endogenous compounds, is very useful for calculating the PMI (and sometimes also the causes of death), even if further studies are needed. The characteristics of VH make it an optimal biological sample for the determination of PMI, given its aqueous constitution and low cellularity, compared to other biological samples, such as blood, being partly protected from post-mortem alterations and bacterial contamination. $K+$ and $NH3$ significantly increase after death, while $Na +$ and Cl-decrease slightly. The slight increase in magnesium lactate, aminoacids and creatinine needs further study. $K+$, $Na+$, $Cl-$ and aminoacids are therefore strongly related to PMI, while $Mg+$, $Cl-$ and lactate are weakly related to PMI. No correlation was found between glucose decrease and PMI, or between creatinine increase and PMI.

Other Authors [49] reviewed 26 publications that provided substantial evidence on structural changes within the eye in determining the PMI, identifying the following application areas: reduction of intraocular pressure; temperature of the eyeball; changes in pupil diameter; corneal thickness and opacity; alterations of the lens; changes in the retina; segmentation of retinal vessels. The major limitations of the studies examined were represented by the use of small case studies, by the absence of a solid statistical methodology and by the use of mathematical models valid only under ideal conditions and, finally, by the use only for short PMI. Although different ocular alterations cannot be used to reliably estimate the PMI, studies indicate that they may be promising in the future thanks to the use of new technologies.

All the methods described above, currently in use, are still imprecise to provide an authentic estimate of the PMI. It is therefore necessary to study new methods to better estimate the PMI. The post-mortem modifications of the corpse are therefore used as "indicators" of the PMI, providing in fact only a completely indicative time range. With the development of molecular biology, attempts have been made to estimate PMI by evaluating the degradation pattern of biological markers (DNA, RNA and Proteins). DNA is shown to be unshakable in the long post-mortem phases, RNA is much more labile in nature and sensitive to degradation in a tissue-specific way. Thus, recently some Authors provided a review that mainly focuses on potential use of RNA markers in estimation of PMI [50]. For this review, the systematic evaluation of 47 studies were executed according to the default inclusion and exclusion criteria. There have been many attempts made by forensic scholars to find out the methods of estimating the PMI accurately, but those methods were based on conventional and established approach. In this recent review, Sangwan et al. [50] reported the use of RNA, DNA and protein degradation for PMI estimation. Many studies have been carried out to find a more accurate and reliable method for estimating the PMI, but currently none can provide an accurate estimate of the PMI. The degradation of DNA nucleic acids appears to be time-correlated such that it is useful for estimating the PMI over long time periods. However, several ante-mortem and post-mortem factors, including environmental conditions, significantly affect DNA degradation. Studies have so far focused on animal models. Then, the development of the multiparametric mathematical model based on DNA degradation has not been able to evaluate the error with a known PMI. Comparatively, the contribution of RNA degradation with molecular approaches in estimating PMI has revealed great potential but is not yet used in forensic practice. Among the studies on RNA degradation based mainly on animal models, only the multiparametric mathematical model is the most reliable method for estimating PMI.

Another new method for estimating PMI is that based on protein degradation. Experimental studies have been conducted on four animal tissues: lungs, kidneys, bones, and skeletal muscles (the only rare, albeit of high quality, performed on human tissue and in the forensic field).

One of the major limitations, in addition to the almost exclusive use of the animal model and obviously not in the forensic field, is the use of biomarkers that are difficult to use on humans.

Certainly, the future will focus on the combination of different methods, also considering the influence of environmental factors in the estimation of the PMI.

Ultimately, further studies on human samples and tissues are needed to better understand the usefulness of such methods. Despite numerous advances in PMI estimation, the inaccuracies observed in these methods require further research effort. In the future, the development of more reliable and cheaper techniques will change the course of forensic science also in the determination of PMI.

It is essential that researchers turn to innovative techniques that produce fast and reliable results, also to obtain validation and acceptance not only in the forensic scientific community but also (and above all) in the courtrooms.

7. The future

A European survey [51] showed that different countries has national autopsy guidelines; the most common protocols concern violent or sudden deaths, mass disasters, and medical negligence.

In the future innovative robotized and advanced microscopy systems and techniques will be utilized, finding their application in the medico legal field, by perfecting and standardizing the autopsy methodology, and achieving a more precise identification of natural and traumatic pathologies.

For improving accuracy and efficiency, the forensic autopsy will performed with a robotic system, using different methods (photogrammetry, optical surface scanning, tissue, or liquid sampling image-guided).

Atomic force microscopy (a high-resolution scanning probe microscopy with production 3-D images), will allow the study of biological macromolecules for the evaluation of PMI.

The direct tissue analysis by MALDI-IMS and SALDI, used for the identification, analysis, spatial profiling and quantification of drugs, heavy metals, proteins, peptides, and metabolites, will increase diagnostic potential and reduce analysis time in forensic cases.

Furthermore, MSI will enable to define tissue types by chemical composition rather than structure, revealing how macromolecules, such as proteins, peptides, nuclei acids, metabolites and xenobiotics are spatially distributed within a given sample. SALDI will be able to detection of small molecules and MSI will promise more sophisticated extensions to forensic applications, including cause of death and PMI identification, by observing the post-mortem decay of metabolites in cells, and the detection and distribution of xenobiotics in tissues.

8. Conclusions

The technological innovation of the medico legal sciences, begun at the end of the 20th century and continuing into the new millennium, has led to the need for an interdisciplinary approach in the execution of the necroscopic ascertainment. In this way the medico legal sciences will be able to identify and describe injuries that could be difficult to objectify and to respond to specific forensic problems, such as the determination of the post-mortem interval, the identification of wound vitality, the reconstruction of the chronology of injuries, or the timing of natural diseases. In particular, the involvement and the integration of multiple specialists such as the forensic pathologist, geneticist, toxicologist, radiologist, anthropologist, microbiologist, and entomologist has become of fundamental importance.

The traditional autopsy is and will probably remain an essential way to investigate the death, despite enormous technological developments and the consequent future prospect of a robotic or virtual autopsy, with the aid of micro- and nanotechnologies.

Therefore, it remains today valid L.S. King affirmed in 1965: it is a mistake to assume that mere autopsy can advance medical science; in fact, scientific progress in the medical field does not depend on the autopsy but on the person who is performing it; so it is important not only (or not so much) the number of autopsies that are performed, but how they are performed, it being essential that the data provided by the autopsies are profitably used, through *"people who have imagination, originality, tenacity, mental acuity"*, but above all adequate and profound scientific preparation, without which the observed data are completely useless [52].

Then, it will not only be necessary that the Forensic Pathology Services are certified and accredited, but also all the specialists involved in the necroscopic ascertainment, from the forensic pathologist to experts such as the radiologist, the toxicologist, the geneticist, thus ensuring a high-quality of the services in the forensic field.

The critical issues that most affect post-mortem forensic evaluation is above all the lack of evidence in scientific knowledge.

The scientific evolution of forensic research will benefit from the omics, bio-analytical, and imaging sciences. In this way, the increased accuracy of the various forensic disciplines will be oriented towards the elaboration of specific *"algorithms"*, able to weigh the value of *"evidence"* placed at the disposal of the *"justice system"* as truth and proof.

Conflict of interest

The authors declare no conflict of interest.

Author details

Massimo Montisci*, Giovanni Cecchetto and Guido Viel
Department of Cardio-Thoraco-Vascular Sciences and Public Health, Section of Legal Medicine, University of Padova, Padova, Italy

*Address all correspondence to: massimo.montisci@unipd.it

References

[1] King LS, Meehan MC. A history of the autopsy. A review. The American Journal of Pathology. 1973;**73**:514-544

[2] Burton JL, Underwood J. Clinical, educational, and epidemiological value of autopsy. Lancet. 2007;**369**:1471-1480

[3] Wood MJ, Guha AK. Declining clinical autopsy rates versus increasing medicolegal autopsy rates in Halifax, Nova Scotia. Archives of Pathology & Laboratory Medicine. 2001;**125**:924-930

[4] De Cock KM, Zielinski-Gutiérrez E, Lucas SL. Learning from the dead. The New England Journal of Medicine. 2019;**381**(20):1889-1891

[5] Snenghi R, Bonvicini B, Scrivano S, Montisci M. The decline and misuse of medical autopsy: Clinical-scientific, medical-legal and ethical implications. Rivista Italiana di Medicina Legale. 2016;**3**:1293-1304

[6] Cecchetto G, Bajanowski T, Cecchi R, Favretto D, Grabherr S, Ishikawa T, et al. Back to the future- part 1 the medico-legal autopsy from ancient civilization to the post-genomic era. International Journal of Legal Medicine. 2017;**31**:1069-1083

[7] Bajanowski T, Vennemann MM. Infanticide. In: Madea B, editor. Handbook of Forensic Medicine. Chichester: Wiley-Blackwell; 2014. pp. 504-515

[8] Bajanowski T, Vege A, Byard RW, et al. Sudden infant death syndrome (SIDS) – Standardised investigations and classification: Recommendations. Forensic Science International. 2007;**165**:129-143

[9] Lignitz E, Kernbach-Wighton G, Henn V. Death during pregnancy. In: Madea B, editor. Handbook of Forensic Medicine. Chichester: Wiley-Blackwell; 2014. pp. 516-524

[10] Pedal I, Moosmayer A, Mallach HJ, Oehmichen M. Air embolism or putrefaction? Gas analysis findings and their interpretation. Zeitschrift für Rechtsmedizin. 1987;**99**:151-167

[11] Beh P. Sexual homicide. In: Madea B, editor. Handbook of Forensic Medicine. Chichester: Wiley-Blackwell; 2014. pp. 539-541

[12] Ferrara SD, Baccino E, Bajanowski T, et al. Malpractice and medical liability. European guidelines on methods of ascertainment and criteria of evaluation. International Journal of Legal Medicine. 2013;**127**:545-557

[13] Brinkmann B. Harmonization of medico-legal autopsy rules. Committee of Ministers. Council of Europe. International Journal of Legal Medicine. 1999;**113**:1-14

[14] Schaffner M. Investigations on the histology and metallization following electric influences on the skin. Deutsche Zeitschrift für die Gesamte Gerichtliche Medizin. 1965;**56**:269-280

[15] Hopkinson DA. The use of Giemsa stain to demonstrate histologically the extent of altered striated muscle around bullet wounds. The Journal of Pathology and Bacteriology. 1964;**87**:63-69

[16] Janssen W. Forensic Histopathology. Berlin, Heidelberg: Springer-Verlag; 1977

[17] Dettmeyer RB. Forensic Histopathology. Fundamentals and Perspectives. Berlin, Heidelberg: Springer Verlag; 2011

[18] Singh S, Abraham JL, Raasch F, Wolf P, Bloor CM. Diagnosis of early human myocardial ischemic damage with electron probe microanalysis. The American Journal of Forensic Medicine and Pathology. 1983;**4**(1):85-91

[19] Ryvarden G. Problems in the determination of gunshot distance by means of the scanning electron microscope at distances over 1 meter. Beiträge zur Gerichtlichen Medizin. 1976;**34**:179-184

[20] Torre C, Varetto L. Dermal surface in electric and thermal injuries. Observations by scanning electron microscopy. The American Journal of Forensic Medicine and Pathology. 1986;**7**(2):151-158

[21] Grellner W, Madea B. Pulmonary micromorphology in fatal strangulations. Forensic Science International. 1994;**67**:109-125

[22] Turillazzi E, Karch SB, Neri M, Pomara C, Riezzo I, Fineschi V. Confocal laser scanning microscopy. Using new technology to answer old questions in forensic investigations. International Journal of Legal Medicine. 2008;**122**:173-177

[23] Thompson TJ, Inglis J. Differentiation of serrated and non-serrated blades from stab marks in bone. International Journal of Legal Medicine. 2009;**123**:129-135

[24] Bortolotti F, Tagliaro F, Manetto G. Objective diagnosis of drowning by the "diatom test" - a critical review. Forensic Science Review. 2004;**16**:135-148

[25] Viel G, Cecchetto G, Fabbri LD, Furlan C, Ferrara SD, Montisci M. Forensic application of ESEM and XRF-EDS techniques to a fatal case of sodium phosphate enema intoxication. International Journal of Legal Medicine. 2009;**123**:345-350

[26] Brown H, Cauchi DM, Holden JL, Allen FC, Cordner S, Thatcher P. Image analysis of gunshot residue on entry wounds. II–A statistical estimation of firing range. Forensic Science International. 1999;**100**:179-186

[27] Cecchi R, Sestili C, Prosperini G, et al. Markers of mechanical asphyxia: Immunohistochemical study on autoptic lung tissues. International Journal of Legal Medicine. 2014;**128**:117-125

[28] Muciaccia B, Sestili C, De Grossi S, Vestri A, Cipolloni L, Cecchi R. Are mast cells implicated in asphyxia? International Journal of Legal Medicine. 2016;**130**:153-161

[29] Cecchi R, Bajanowski T, Kahl B. Wiegand P.CMV-DNA detection in parenchymatous organs in cases of SIDS. International Journal of Legal Medicine. 1995;**107**:291-295

[30] United Nations Manual on the Effective Prevention and Investigation of Extra-Legal Arbitrary and Summary Executions, IV. Model autopsy protocol. Available form: https://tavaana.org/sites/default/files/UN_Manual_on_the_Effective_Prevention_and_Investigation%5B1%5D.pdf

[31] Montisci M, El Mazloum R, Cecchetto G, et al. Anabolic androgenic steroids abuse and cardiac death in athletes: Morphological and toxicological findings in four fatal cases. Forensic Science International. 2012;**217**:e13-e18

[32] Cecchetto G, Viel G, Amagliani A, Boscolo-Berto R, Fais P, Montisci M. Histological diagnosis of myocardial sarcoidosis in a fatal fall from a height. Journal of Forensic Sciences. 2011;**56**(Suppl 1):S255-S258

[33] Cecchetto G, Viel G, Cecchetto A, Kusstatscher S, Montisci M. Fatal splenic rupture following Heimlich maneuver: Case report and literature review. The American Journal of Forensic Medicine and Pathology. 2011;**32**:169-171

[34] Ferrara SD, Cecchetto G, Cecchi R, Favretto D, Grabherr S, Ishikawa T, et al. Back to the future - part 2 post-mortem assessment and evolutionary role of the bio-Medicolegal sciences. International Journal of Legal Medicine. 2017;**131**:1085-1101

[35] Dirnhofer R, Jackowski C, Vock P, Potter K, Thali MJ. VIRTOPSY: Minimally invasive, imaging-guided virtual autopsy. Radiographics. 2006;**26**:1305-1333

[36] Jolibert M, Cohen F, Bartoli C, et al. Postmortem CT-angiography: Feasibility of US-guided vascular access. Journal de Radiologie. 2011;**92**:446-449

[37] Brough AL, Morgan B, Rutty GN. Postmortem computed tomography (PMCT) and disaster victim identification. La Radiologia Medica. 2015;**120**:866-873

[38] Borowska-Solonynko A, Solonynko B. The use of 3D computed tomography reconstruction in medico-legal testimony regarding injuries in living victims—Risks and benefits. Journal of Forensic and Legal Medicine 2015; 30: 9-13.

[39] Giorgetti A, Giraudo C, Viero A, Bisceglia M, Lupi A, Fais P, et al. Radiological investigation of gunshot wounds: A systematic review of published evidence. International Journal of Legal Medicine. 2019;**133**(4):1149-1158

[40] Roberts IS, Benamore RE, Benbow EW, et al. Post-mortem imaging as an alternative to autopsy in the diagnosis of adult deaths: A validation study. Lancet. 2012;**379**:136-142

[41] Saunders SL, Morgan B, Raj V, Robinson CE, Rutty GN. Targeted post-mortem computed tomography cardiac angiography: Proof of concept. International Journal of Legal Medicine. 2011;**125**:609-616

[42] Fais P, Cecchetto G, Boscolo-Berto R, Toniolo M, Viel G, Miotto D, et al. Morphometric analysis of stab wounds by MSCT and MRI after the instillation of contrast medium. La Radiologia Medica. 2016;**121**:494-501

[43] Blitz AM, Aygun N, Herzka DA. Invited commentary: The rise of microradiology. Radiographics. 2015;**35**: 1091-1093

[44] Fais P, Giraudo C, Viero A, Miotto D, Bortolotti F, Tagliaro F, et al. Micro computed tomography features of laryngeal fractures in a case of fatal manual strangulation. Legal Medicine (Tokyo, Japan). 2016;**18**:85-89

[45] Mangin P, Bonbled F, Vali M, et al. European Council of Legal Medicine (ECLM) accreditation of forensic pathology services in Europe. International Journal of Legal Medicine. 2015;**129**:395-403

[46] Examiners NAoM. NAME Inspection and Accreditation Checklist for Autopsy Services. 2014. Revised 2019. Available from: https://www.thename.org

[47] Madea B, Henssge C. General remark on estimating the time since death. In: Madea B, editor. Estimation of the Time since Death. CPR Press: Taylor & Francis Group; 2016. pp. 1-4

[48] Pigaiani N, Bertaso A, De Palo EF, Bortolotti F, Tagliaro F. Vitreous humor endogenous compounds analysis for

post-mortem forensic investigation. Forensic Science International. 2020;**310**:110235

[49] De-Giorgio F, Grassi S, d'Aloja E, Pascali VL. Post-mortem ocular changes and time since death: Scoping review and future perspective. Legal Medicine (Tokyo, Japan). 2021;**50**:101862

[50] Sangwan A, Singh SP, Singh P, Gupta OP, Manas A, Gupta S. Role of molecular techniques in PMI estimation: An update. Journal of Forensic and Legal Medicine. 2021;**83**:102251

[51] Ferrara SD, Bajanowski T, Cecchi R, Boscolo-Berto R, Viel G. Bio-medicolegal scientific research in Europe: A comprehensive bibliometric overview. International Journal of Legal Medicine. 2011;**125**:393-402

[52] King LS. Of autopsies. Maryland State Medical Journal. 1965;**14**:59-60

Chapter 4

Medicolegal Autopsy

Nisha Goyal and Anil Garg

Abstract

The word autopsy is formed from two Greek words, Autos and Optos. The meaning of the word Autos is self and the word Optos is seen. Thus, autopsy means seeing of self. An autopsy is of two types. Medicolegal Autopsy and Histopathological or Clinical Autopsy. In this chapter, we mainly focus on the Medicolegal autopsy, what is the aim of the autopsy. What are the prerequisites of the autopsy? Where medicolegal autopsy can be carried out? Who can carry out the autopsy. What are the different incisions of doing a medico-legal autopsy? We also discuss which viscera are to persevere in different autopsy procedures and which trace elements are to be collected in common medicolegal autopsies. How viscera and trace evidence collected from the dead body are preserved. We will also discuss, in brief, the preservatives used.

Keywords: clinical autopsy, postmortem examination, viscera, preservatives, dissection, evidence, weapon

1. Introduction

The word Autopsy is formed from two Greek words, Autos and Optos. The meaning of the word Autos is self and the word Optos is seen. Thus, autopsy means seeing of self. It is also commonly known as postmortem examination. An autopsy is of two types:

1. Medicolegal Autopsy/Forensic Autopsy.

2. Histopathological Autopsy/Clinical Autopsy.

Medicolegal Autopsy is done in deaths due to unnatural causes and in natural cases also, where the cause of death is not certain or brings dead cases [1]. The aim and objective of the medicolegal autopsy are to help the law enforcement agencies to ascertain the identity of the deceased, cause of death, type of weapon used, Time since death, manner of death and to collect any trace evidence. The registered medical practitioners are only legally allowed to do the autopsy in India in the medicolegal case at the request of the investigating officer, along with inquest papers at the authorized place only. The consent of relatives is not required. However, relatives are required for the identification of the deceased before starting a postmortem examination. After completing the postmortem, the body of the deceased is handed over to the police/Investigating officer along with numbered and initial inquest papers and a medicolegal autopsy report. While, in the Clinical Autopsy, the autopsy is to be done by a Pathologist after taking the consent of the relatives for autopsy and investigation if any is required. Before starting a clinical autopsy, it should be insured or verified that it is not a medicolegal case. It is done at the request of clinical doctors and after authorization from the head of the hospital, to know the disease process which was going on in the deceased body, to further augment the knowledge of medicine. The pathologist may or may not share the autopsy report with the relatives. In a medicolegal autopsy, the background information is minimal, maybe distorted or non-scientific as per the knowledge available with the investigating police official while in the histopathological autopsy, the detailed events of disease, case sheets made by well-educated staff are available. The report of the medicolegal autopsy will be crossed by a defense lawyer in the court of law while the histopathological autopsy is crossed by peer review in case discussion meetings [2].

The Medicolegal Autopsy is studied under the following heads

- Preliminary Examination of Inquest Papers.
- Gross/External Examination of the body
- Internal examination of the body.
  - Skin incisions
  - Methods of removal of organs
  - Samples to be collected
- Preservatives used for various samples

2. Preliminary examination of inquest papers

Medicolegal Autopsy is done on the orders of legal authorities like Police, Magistrate, or Coroner. In India, in most cases, a Medicolegal autopsy is ordered by the police, Hence known as Police Inquest. In a few medicolegal cases like dowry death, custodial death under armed forces, etc. are ordered by Magistrate, Hence, it is known as Magistrate Inquest. In the western world, Inquests are done by the coroner also. Hence, it is known as Coroner Inquest.

Inquest means Inquiry or Investigation. The officer who is authorized to do an inquest is known as Investigation Officer. The investigating officer may be a Police official, Magistrate, or Coroner depending upon the case to be investigated according to local laws. A medicolegal autopsy is usually done in sudden, unexplained, or unnatural deaths. In India, the investigating officer requests a Registered Medical officer (RMP) with an application for autopsy along with inquest papers. In India, an investigation is done by Police officials under sections 174 and Magistrate under Section 176 of the Criminal Procedure Code, 1973 to inquire in cases of suicide and suspicious deaths whereas, under Section 174 [3], deaths related to dowry or cruelty by in-laws were investigated [3].

After completion of the investigation report by the Police officer, he/she will have to submit an Inquest report in Form 25.35 [1] A, B, C for natural causes, violence, and poisoning cases respectively. The inquest report should mention the apparent cause of death, description of any mark or marks of violence which may be found on the body, and description of the alleged weapon used. The Inquest report should contain the plan of the scene of death, the inventory of the clothing, etc. A list of the articles on and with the body, a list of the articles sent for medical examination, if any, and a copy of police information (PI) from the Hospital, Hospital record along with a death summary [4].

3. Gross/external examination of the body

Before starting the postmortem examination, the registered medical practitioner (Medical officer) note down the preliminary data related to the deceased in the computerized format like name, father name, age sex, the residence, report number, date, name of investigating officer with belt number and police station, names, and signatures of two relatives who identify the body of deceased on autopsy table before starting of postmortem examination.

Gross examination of the deceased is one of the important steps in doing an autopsy. In medicolegal cases, like a road traffic accident, homicide, suicide, burns, vitriolage, firearm, etc., gross examination gives valuable information to augment internal examination. During the gross or external examination, we record the following parameters from the body of the deceased.

a. Height

b. Weight

c. Clothes

d. Skin (injuries, tattoos, moles, and any disease)

e. Eyes (Injuries, Tardieu spots, Hemorrhages)

f. Mouth (externally) including lips

g. Nose (injury, deformity, blood, etc.)

h. Face, Ears, and neck (injuries, nail marks, ligature, injection marks)

i. Palpate Chest, abdomen and testis

j. Back of the body and lower and upper limbs (injuries, nail marks, ligature, injection marks)

After noting down the above parameters, photography should be done before removing or handling the body. Clothes are removed from the body with most precaution. All the clothes should be preserved and photographed separately. It should be ensured that any cuts, and tears on clothes are not distorted while removing the clothes from the body. In case of homicide and cases where the investigating officer requested for sealing of the clothes, it should be labeled with the postmortem number, signed along with the date, and sealed in a packet with seals as specified, with a proper label, signature, and stamped for finally handing over to the investigating officer. Any trace evidence recovered during removal of clothes from the body like nails parts, firearm projectile lying loose should be preserved separately in a packet, labeled, sealed, signed and stamped, and handed over to investigating officer after completion of autopsy after taking receipt to maintain the chain of custody of the evidence.

4. Internal examination of the body

After doing a gross or external examination and removal of clothes from the body of the deceased, Again examination of the deceased body is to be done to look for any injuries, biological material like semen, saliva, and any foreign body. With Gross examination, we had already made a preliminary road map to proceed further. There are three cavities in the body, Abdominal or peritoneal cavity, Thoracic cavity, and cranial cavity. Depending upon the nature of the case, we open the cavity where we see more injuries. But as a routine, we open the skull first followed by the abdomen and chest. After opening the skull first, all the blood was drained out from the neck. Thus, we got a clear bloodless view of neck tissues. So, the case of asphyxia like hanging and strangulation is well appreciated.

But on gross examination, we found injuries to the abdomen and thorax, then we opened the abdomen and thorax first followed by the cranial cavity.

5. Skin incisions used for opening cavities during autopsy

A cranial incision is the most common incision given on the scalp starting from the mastoid process of one side of the skull going superiorly passing through the vertex of the cranial cavity and ending on the mastoid process of another side. The scalp is reflected up to the frontal eminence on the front and the occipital protuberance on the back of the skull. Then the cranial vault is opened with a skull opening machine by giving a V or Z-shaped incision on the outside of the skull. V and Z-shaped cut in the cranial vault help in a tight fit on stitching the scalp after placing the cranial vault.

There are mainly three conventional skin incisions used in most of the world on the thorax and chest while doing the autopsy. These are as follows:-

5.1 I-shaped incision

This incision is widely used while opening the abdominal and thoracic cavity. I-shaped incision starts from just below the chin and reaches up to the pubic symphysis, curving around the umbilicus laterally. The umbilicus is left as such to maintain the cosmetic effect and technically, it consists of dense fibrous tissue, it is difficult to cut through it and later on difficult to stitch (**Figures 1–3**).

5.2 Y-shaped incision

This incision is the next common incision given while opening the abdominal and thoracic cavity. The Y-shaped incision starts from just below the mastoid process on both sides as two limbs of Y, descends anterior-inferiorly and meets in the midline at the level of the suprasternal notch and then proceeds downwards up to the pubic symphysis, curving around the umbilicus laterally similar to I-shaped skin incision.

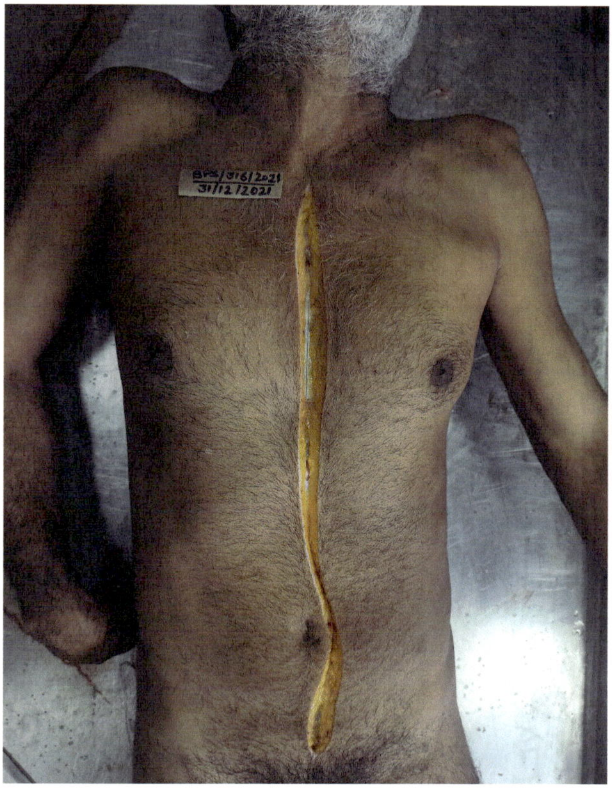

Figure 1.
Showed I-shaped incision on the front of the body of the deceased in the supine position. The figure showed an incision starting from the suprasternal notch of Manubrium going downwards in midline curving around the umbilicus up to symphysis pubis in the supine position. This incision is extended upwards up to the chin in the midline to complete the I-shaped Incision.

This type of incision is used in medicolegal cases of autopsy where layer by layer dissection of the neck is required to demonstrate neck injuries as well as ligature marks e.g. In asphyxia due to neck compression-like Hanging, Strangulation, etc. In the neck region, the large neck veins are present superficially. So, there are chances of artifactual air embolism (**Figures 4–6**).

5.3 Modified Y-shaped incision

This incision is the third most common incision given while opening the abdominal and thoracic cavity. It is usually given in females and VIP cases, where the body is to be kept for the last homage to the public to avoid disfigurement and public outrage. Modified Y-shaped incision starts from the acromion on both sides of the shoulder, then descends downwards curving the outer shoulder joint anteriorly, reaching to the anterior axillary folds and curving below both breasts and meets in the midline at the xiphisternum level and then proceeds downwards up to the pubic symphysis, curving around the umbilicus laterally (**Figures 7–10**).

There are few more incisions, other than these three conventional incisions which are used by different autopsy surgeons as per convenience.

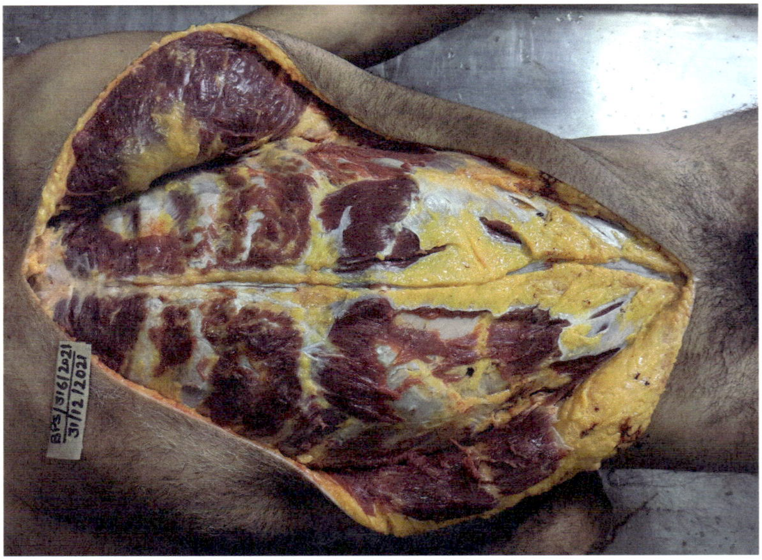

Figure 2.
Showed I-shaped incision on the body of the deceased in the supine position. The figure showed I-shaped incision starting from the suprasternal notch of the manubrium to symphysis pubis along with soft tissue dissection to raise the flaps for further dissection.

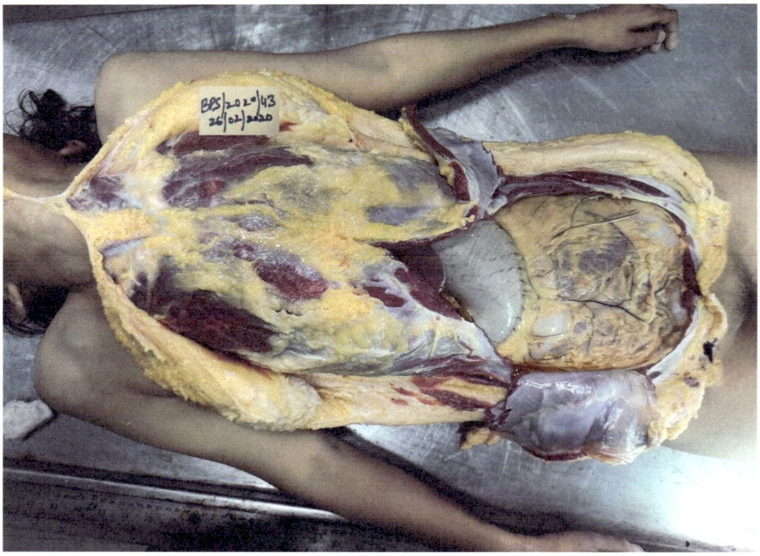

Figure 3.
Showed I-shaped incision on the body of the deceased in the supine position. The figure showed I-shaped incision starting from the suprasternal notch of the manubrium to symphysis pubis to raise the flaps of skin on either side of the abdomen and then opening of the abdominal cavity in the midline and below the subcostal margins and then retracting the abdominal muscular flaps to either side for the internal dissection of the abdominal organs.

5.4 Fourth incision

All the conventional incisions as described above are on the front of the neck, chest, and abdomen, Hence, it was difficult to tell about injuries on the back of

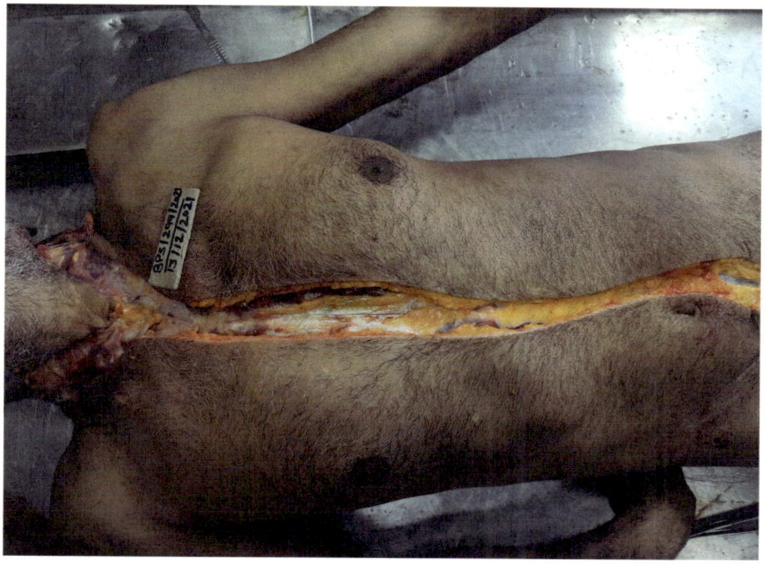

Figure 4.
Showed a Y-shaped skin incision on the body of the deceased in the supine position. The Y-shaped incision started from just below the mastoid process on both sides as two limbs of the Y, descends anterior-inferiorly and meets in the midline at the level of the suprasternal notch and then proceeds downwards up to the pubic symphysis, curving around the umbilicus laterally similar to I-shaped skin incision.

the neck, chest, and abdomen. In India, It is also routine practice to replace all the dissected organs in the abdominal cavity and thoracic cavity in one single incision as mentioned above. So, there are chances of seepage of the blood from this single incision. So, to overcome this problem, another incision named the fourth incision as per the author [5] was advised. The incision is also cosmetically better appealing to immediate legal heirs before the last rituals. For the anterior approach, the body is kept in a supine position with a block under the shoulder to extend the neck. The incision is started from one side of the mastoid process to the other side passing through the vertex in the coronal plane. The scalp is reflected up to occipital protuberance in the back and frontal eminence in front, thus exposing the skull bone for further dissection. The incisions on both sides of the mastoid process are extended downwards up to the acromion process and pass in front of the chest outside the shoulder joint to the midaxillary line below the axilla and then further extended to the anterior superior iliac spine, then turning to the middle along with inguinal ligaments to meet each other in midline. Now, the flap is raised by superficial dissection up to the root of the neck furthering up to the lower border of the mandible. Then, the abdominal cavity is opened by giving a midline incision. The dissection is further preceded, as usual, then again, the body is stitched in the midline and then skin incision is stitched starting from the inguinal region on both sides and then sideways. To do dissection on the posterior side of the body, it is kept in a prone position with a block under the chest to raise it and flex the neck. Now again, the incision is extended from the right acromion posteriorly, curving the outer side of the shoulder on both sides reaching up to the midaxillary line, and further extended to the anterior superior iliac spine on both sides. Now the scalp flap raised to occipital protuberance is further extended through the neck, back of the chest, and lower back and raised inferiorly. Now, the underlying dissection was done. The stitching

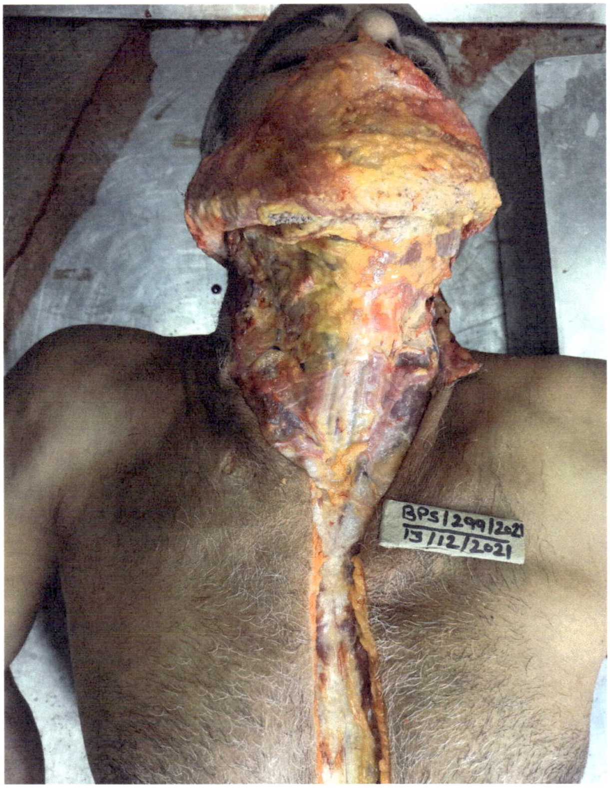

Figure 5.
Showed a Y-shaped skin incision on the neck and the chest of the deceased in the supine position. The flap of the skin is retracted superiorly up to the level of the chin and the lower border of the mandible as a V-shaped flap. This will give a clear field for dissection at the neck.

on the back is done after replacing the flap superiorly with an anteriorly replaced scalp flap. Afterward, later sidewall stitching is done.

Few authors also advised fifth or another incision [6] to reduce the time taken for suturing and disfigurement of the body of the deceased. The body is kept in a supine position with a block under the back of the chest to extend the neck. This incision starts from the right mastoid process and goes towards the left mastoid process in the coronal plane on the scalp. From the right mastoid process, the incision moves on the front of the neck to reach the left incision on the left mastoid process just two fingerbreadths inferior to the lower border of the chin. The incision from the right mastoid process goes down on the lateral side of the neck up to the right acromion process. Then from the right acromion process, the incision is curved in front of the medial end of the right shoulder to reach the level of the mid-axillary line of the fourth rib, from here it goes down up to the right anterior superior iliac spine, then move towards the left side on the front of the abdomen near inguinal ligament and reaches up to the left anterior superior iliac spine. Now, dissection of the underlying tissues is done horizontally to raise the flap of skin on the front of the chest and abdomen. Now, to open the abdominal cavity, a muscular incision is started just above the right anterior superior iliac spine which extends towards the left anterior superior iliac spine along the inguinal canals, then extends superiorly up to the level of tenth

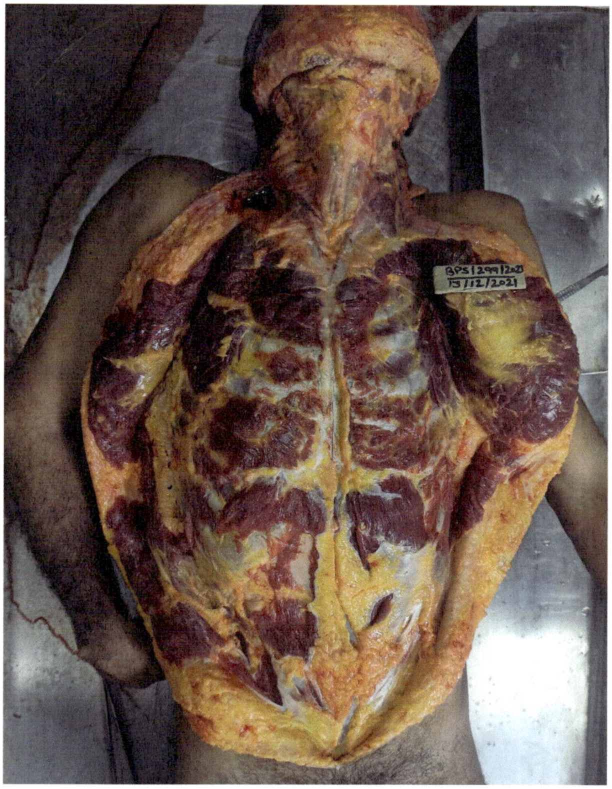

Figure 6.
Showed a Y-shaped incision on the body of the deceased in the supine position. The figure showed Y-shaped incision starting from each mastoid process and merging in the midline at the level of the suprasternal notch of the manubrium further proceeded to symphysis pubis curving the umbilicus along with the soft tissue dissection to raise the flaps on the front of the chest, abdomen and neck area for further dissection.

rib costal cartilage and then again extends towards right side till right costal margin near the midaxillary line. After this incision, the flap of the muscular abdominal wall is raised towards the right side. After doing dissection, the flap is replaced without stitching and then the body is stitched starting from the skin incision near the left anterior superior iliac spine to the right mastoid process. If dissection is required on the back of the body, then the body is kept in a prone position with a block below the chest to flex the neck. Starting from the incision made in an anterior approach, the incision is extended posteriorly on the outer side of the right shoulder from the right acromion process up to the right mid-axillary line meeting the incision already given in the anterior approach. From the anterior superior iliac spine, the incision has to be extended along the upper convex borders of the buttocks from the right to the left anterosuperior spine. Now dissection is done tangentially and the flap on the backside of the chest and lower back is raised on the left side separating the underlying muscles and body attachments after dissection of the back, the skin is sutured from the left anterosuperior spine to the right acromion process. The length of this incision is less than the fourth incision as discussed above, but more than the conventional I, Y, and Modified Y-shaped incisions, and thus suturing can be done early as compared to the fourth incision. However, similar to the fourth Incision, it is cosmetically appealing and avoids seepage of contents as occurred in the conventional skin incisions.

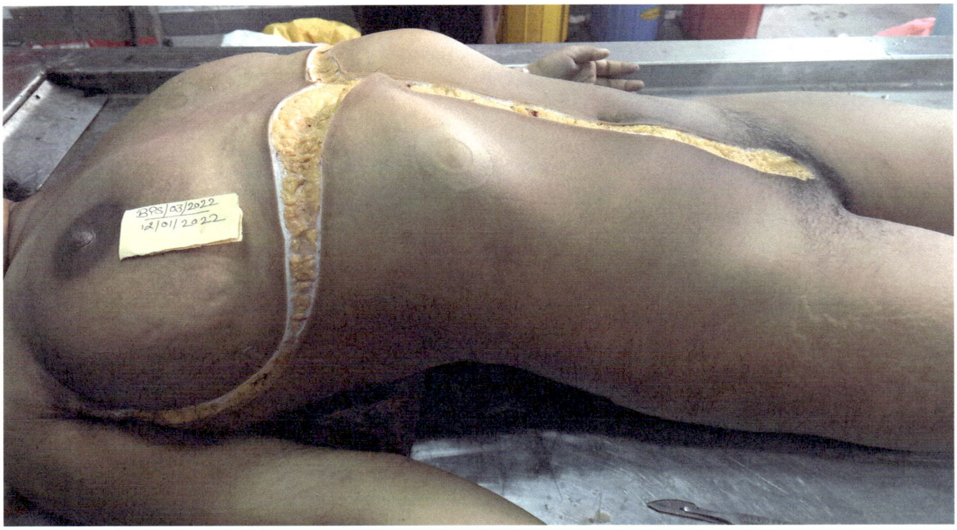

Figure 7.
Showed a Modified Y-shaped skin incision on the body of the female deceased. Modified Y-shaped incision starts from the acromion, then descends curving around the outer side of the shoulder, then reaching anterior axillary folds and curving below both breasts and meets in the midline at the xiphisternum level and then proceeds downwards up to the pubic symphysis, curving around the umbilicus laterally.

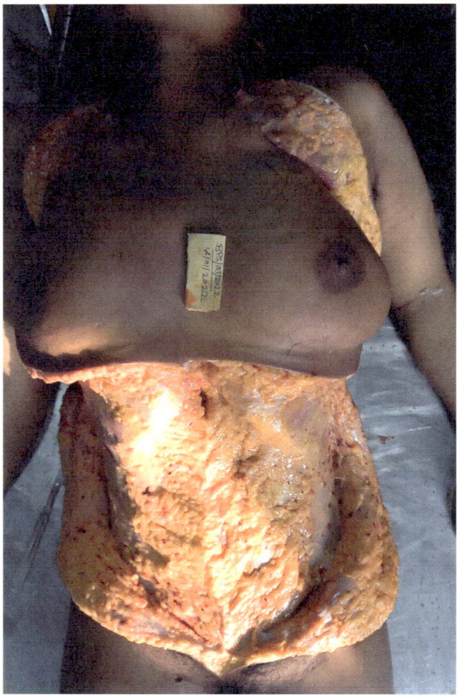

Figure 8.
Showed a Modified Y-shaped skin incision with underlying soft tissue dissection on the body of the female deceased. Modified Y-shaped incision along with underlying soft tissue dissection is done to raise the abdominal flaps and mammary flaps.

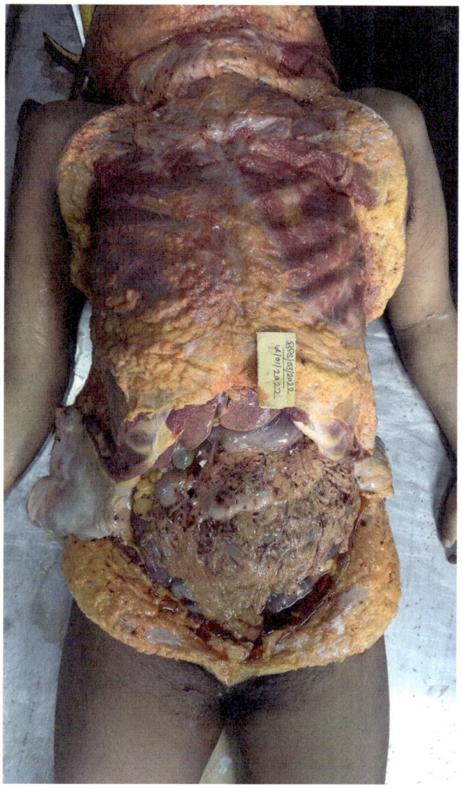

Figure 9.
Showed a Modified Y-shaped incision with underlying soft tissue and abdominal wall dissection on the body of the female deceased. Modified Y-shaped incision with underlying soft tissue dissection is done to raise the abdominal flaps and mammary flaps. The abdominal wall is opened in the midline and below the sub-costal cartilage to raise the abdominal wall flaps on each side of the abdomen to open the abdominal cavity.

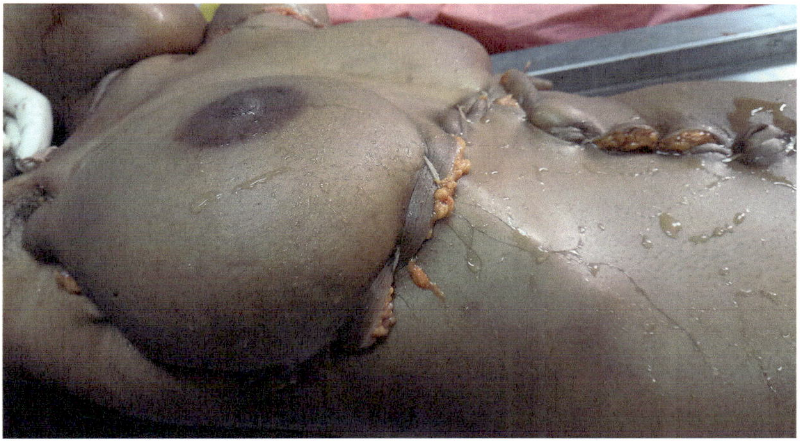

Figure 10.
Showed stitched modified Y-shaped incisions on the body of the female deceased. The Modified Y-shaped incision is stitched to retain the anatomical appearance of the body of the deceased. The neck and face are cosmetically preserved due to dissection of underlying tissue after raising the flaps.

6. Methods of removal of organs during autopsy

There are four conventional methods known to remove organs from the body of the deceased during autopsy [7].

6.1 Rokitansky's technique or method of removal of organs

As the name suggests, this technique was devised by a German pathologist named Carl Rakitansky (1804–78). In this technique, Autopsy dissection is done in situ. Advantages: Easy to do in infected bodies as well in children. Disadvantage: This technique is difficult to perform in adults.

6.2 Virchow's technique or method of removal of organs

As the name suggests, this technique was performed by a German pathologist named Rudolph Virchow (1821–1902). In this technique, organs are removed one by one and studied as separate entities. Advantages: Easy to study each organ. Disadvantage: The relationship between organs is lost. Thus valuable information may be lost.

6.3 Letulle's technique or method of removal of organs

As the name suggests, this technique was performed by a French pathologist named Maurice Letulle (1853–1929). In this technique, organs are removed together in one mass from tongue to prostate.

Advantages: In this technique, interpersonal relationships are well maintained. Relationships to vessels, lymphatic and nerves are well preserved.

Disadvantage: This is a cumbersome technique and all organs are difficult to manage.

6.4 Ghon's technique or method of removal of organs

As the name suggests, this technique was performed by an Austrian pathologist named Anton Ghon (1866–1936). In this technique, organs are removed in 3 separate blocks. This technique accommodates both Virchow's and Letulles's techniques in one setting. This technique is also known as the Enbloc Method.

Advantages: Since organs are removed in 3 blocs. So, the interrelationship between organs in each block is well maintained. Handling of organs is easy as compared to Letulle's technique where organs are removed en masse.

Disadvantages: Interrelationships are difficult to study if the disease extends across the blocs.

7. Viscera/samples to be collected with preservatives used for medicolegal cases

In Medicolegal cases, various samples are collected depending on the case to case [8].

7.1 Stomach

The entire stomach is tied on above and below the stomach opening and contents are poured into a Jar (preferably a glass jar with a tight lid) by giving an incision at the greater curvature. The stomach wall is inverted and mucosa is examined for congestion, ulceration, and sticky material. The contents of the stomach are also examined for consistency, odor, and color. The stomach and entire contents of the stomach are preserved for detection of poisons in a saturated solution of common salt in suspected common poisons. Rectified spirit is used as a preservative in acid poisoning except for carbolic acid.

7.2 Small intestine and large intestine

Part of the small intestine and large intestine are preserved similar to the stomach as mentioned above in a Jar (preferably a glass jar with a tight lid) for detection of poisons.

7.3 Spleen, kidneys, and liver

Part of the spleen, half of each kidney in the coronal plane, and part of the liver from each lobe or suspected area are also preserved similar to the stomach as mentioned above in a Jar (preferably a glass jar with a tight lid) for detection of poisons. For Microbiological examination, Blood swabs are taken from the spleen. The spleen is kept straight on the autopsy table. The wide base hot sterilized knife is taken and then touched to the spleen twice. This will sterilize the spleen on the outside. Now, the cross incision is given on the sterilized surface of the spleen. The blood swabs are taken from the cuts on the spleen and sent for microbiological examination.

7.4 Gallbladder

The entire gallbladder is preserved and sent for chemical examination along with part of the livers as mentioned above. This is used for the poisons which are excreted through the Biliary System. The Bile can be excreted by giving a cut to the gallbladder wall and collecting bile in the container inserting a needle of the syringe and aspirating bile or collecting bile by squeezing the gallbladder through the cystic duct.

7.5 Blood

After removal of viscera, 10–20 ml of blood should be collected. The femoral vein is the most preferred site for the collection of blood, followed by the iliac vein and Subclavian vein. Never take bloody fluid directly from the heart or scoop it out of thoracic or abdominal cavities. No preservative should be used, when we are sending blood for the detection of common poisons. For Microbiological examination, a Blood culture vial is used to preserve the blood. For Dengue serology and other serological tests, Blood should be preserved in Red Vacutainer. For Alcohol estimation, Blood should be preserved in Sodium fluoride and potassium oxalate solution; else we can also use Phenyl mercuric chloride or Sodium Azide. For blood grouping or DNA/RNA analysis, drops of blood are preserved in an FTA Card [9].

7.6 Anal swabs

These are taken when anal intercourse is suspected. Two sterilized swabs in glass test tubes labeled A and B are taken. A – Swab is taken from deep inside the anal canal. B-Swab is taken from outside the anal canal or as such as control. After taking the swabs, the respective slides are made swabs are kept in respective test tubes and all are kept aside and air-dried, labeled before packaging and sealing for onward transmission.

7.7 Vaginal swabs

These are taken when sexual intercourse is suspected. Two sterilized swabs in glass test tubes labeled A and B are taken. A – Swab is taken from deep inside the vagina preferably posterior fornix. B-Slide is taken from outside the vagina or as such as control. After taking the swabs, the respective slides are made, swabs are kept in respective test tubes and all are kept aside and air-dried, labeled before packaging and sealing for onward transmission.

Both anal and vaginal swabs are preserved for the detection of spermatozoa.

7.8 Saliva/bite marks

In medicolegal cases, if we come across bite marks then we suspect dried saliva. A cotton swab moistened with saline solution is taken and rotated on the bite mark then the swab is kept aside for drying and then kept back in a glass test tube. Saliva is useful in the detection of Blood group (if secretors) and DNA analysis from mucosal cells in saliva.

7.9 Urine

It is usually preserved when we suspect that poison is excreted through urine. The preservative used for Urine is Thymol or Sodium benzoate solution.

7.10 DNA analysis

Long bones are preserved free from skin and muscle tissue preferably in dry ice for DNA Analysis.

7.11 Diatom test

The sternum is preserved to detect diatoms in the bone marrow in suspected cases of drowning.

7.12 Feces

For detection of protozoal and helminthic infestation, 5 to 10 g of feces is collected. In Autopsy cases, it is rarely collected these days.

7.13 CSF

CSF is collected by using a needle and syringe from cisterna magna.

7.14 Vitreous humor

Vitreous Humor is withdrawn from each eye 1 to 5 ml in quantity. It is used to determine the time since death from the potassium etc. level in the vitreous humor [10] and aqueous humor.

For Histopathological examination, the Suspected pathological part of the Lungs, Brain, Kidney, Spleen, Liver, and Skin tissue is collected and sent. These should be preserved in a 10% Formalin solution. The Pieces should be small. Thus formalin can penetrate the tissues quickly and to more areas. Thus the problem of autolysis due to unpreserved tissue is restricted.

8. Conclusions

It is always said that Justice delayed is justice denied. Medico-Legal Autopsy is a process to help law enforcing agencies to understand the cause of death etc., to give justice to the deceased as well as their near and dear ones. So, we should continuously update our knowledge and concepts to help our law enforcement agencies to deliver justice in time.

Acknowledgements

We want to thank open source Intech Publishers and the editor of the book, "Autopsy - What Do We Learn from Corpses?" Who invited us to write a chapter in this book by granting a waiver? We also want to thank all the authors whose articles and literature were referenced to make our knowledge and understanding rich. We are also thankful to the entire staff, especially postgraduate students of the Department of Forensic Medicine, BPS Government Medical College for Women, Gohana, Haryana, India for helping and encouraging us in completing this project in time. This concept of open-source publication is very encouraging. This is our effort to reproduce the work of all the referenced authors and editors in our language for a better understanding of our readers. Thanks.

Conflict of interest

No conflict of interest is present with anybody.

Author details

Nisha Goyal[1] and Anil Garg[2*]

1 Department of Human Anatomy, Rama Medical College Hospital,
Hapur, Uttar Pradesh, India

2 Department of Forensic Medicine and Toxicology, BPS Government Medical College for Women, Gohana, Haryana, India

*Address all correspondence to: anil9637@yahoo.com

References

[1] Nadesan K. The importance of the medico-legal autopsy. The Malaysian Journal of Pathology. 1997;**19**(2):105-109

[2] Kotabagi RB, Charati SC, JD. Clinical autopsy vs medicolegal autopsy. Medical Journal, Armed Forces India. 2005;**61**(3):258-263

[3] Goutam S. Inquest procedure in judicial investigation in India: With Reference to the Proposed New Corner Act. Supreme Law Today. 2010;**6**(133):35-41

[4] The Punjab Police Rules. (As applicable In Haryana State). 1934. Available from: https://haryanapolice.gov.in/pdf/PPR_Volume_III.pdf. [cited 2022 January 15]

[5] Patowary A. The fourth incision: A cosmetic autopsy incision technique. The American Journal of Forensic Medicine and Pathology. 2010;**31**(1):37-41

[6] Kapila P, Gupta R, Raina SK, Sharma AK, Gupta D, Sharma M. Development of a new skin incision for conduct of conventional autopsy. Egyptian Journal of Forensic Sciences. 2018;**8**(54):1-7

[7] Ludwig J. Handbook of Autopsy. 3rd ed. Totowa, New Jersey: Humana Press; 2002. p. 3

[8] Aggrawal A. Textbook of Forensic Medicine and Toxiology. 2nd ed. Kundli, Haryana, India: Avichal Publishing Company; 2021. pp. 140-145

[9] da Cunha SG. FTA cards for preservation of nucleic acids for molecular assays: A review on the use of cytologic/tissue samples. Archives of Pathology & Laboratory Medicine. 2018;**142**(3):308-312

[10] Komura S, Oshiro S. Potassium levels in the aqueous and vitreous humor after death. The Tohoku Journal of Experimental Medicine. 1977;**122**(1):65-68

Chapter 5

Virtopsy: A New Era in Forensic Medico-Legal Autopsies

Pooja Ahuja and Niha Ansari

Abstract

In the field of forensic science, autopsy that is postmortem examination involves a thorough corpse examination done in order to determine the cause and manner of the death by invasive method. With the advancement of technology a new term: "Virtopsy" meaning virtual autopsy employs the application of imaging techniques namely computed tomography (CT) and magnetic resonance imaging (MRI) has proven its advantages in the forensic field. It involves the scanning of dead bodies in a non-invasive manner. It a great alternative to the traditional autopsy as it provides wide-range and systemic examination of the whole body in a less time duration, benefits in diagnosis as well as renders respect to religious sentiments. Method is more specific, sensitive, & precise and accurately reflect soft tissue injuries, organ damage, wound extent, fractures which provides instinctive and powerful court evidence for forensic identification. The chapter will be describing the importance of "Virtopsy" in the field of forensic science and its future scope in forensic crime investigations.

Keywords: forensic science, autopsy, Virtopsy, CT, MRI, 3D scanning

1. Introduction

Traditional autopsy is one of the classical method utilized for the investigation and identification of cause & manner of death. This scientific examination procedure of dead bodies involves complete exposure of the body surface and cavities in order to record the findings which will prove to be useful in establishing the facts pertaining to the circumstances leading to the death of an individual and helping the law enforcement. At the same time gaining consent for the forensic autopsy involves relatives' sentiment or religious belief. Furthermore, some religious and cultural aspects oppose for the autopsy procedure such as Judaism, does not permit the same [1–3]. All these aspects direct the need of a ameliorate autopsy method which overcomes these deterrents and equally prove to be as significant as the traditional method of autopsy. "Virtual Autopsy" or Virtopsy is the new method which is one step towards these advance technology in the field of forensic science.

Virtopsy is a modern method which is scalpel free techniques of performing autopsy using modern imaging and measuring technology [4]. It was coined by Richard Dirnhofer, the former Director of Forensic Medicine, University of Berne's Institute of Forensic Medicine, Switzerland [5]. The virtopsy procedure includes a complete Three-dimensional (3D) surface scanning 3D/computer-aided design photogrammetry, Multi-slice computed tomography (MSCT), Magnetic resonance imaging (MRI) and MRI spectroscopy [6]. It provides a complete inside and outside view of the body in three dimensional way. The vital information such as position and dimensions of injuries or severity of injuries or other pathological conditions can be gather in a digitalize manner, thus facilitating effective assessment of body's condition. It's a promising tool encompassing high scanning and radiographic technology possessing the power and resolution of modern computing, which prove to be useful to investigators, forensic pathologists and doctors [7].

2. Application of Virtopsy in forensic sciences

Virtopsy has shown its wide range of applications in the field of forensic with respect to various aspects such as thanatological investigations, firearms injury, age estimation, fracture estimation, putrefied body identifications, forensic odontology, mass disaster cases, anthropological examinations, drowning cases, skin lesion analyses, charred bodies identification etc.

In drowning cases, determination of whether the drowning is ante-mortem or postmortem and what is the actual cause of death is very significant for the forensic experts. The computed tomography (CT) data reveling evidences about the volume of liquid present in lungs, density and size of the lungs thus helping in identifying the actual cause of death. Levy et al., in 2007 [8] performed the post-mortem computed tomography (PMCT) in drowning cases and first reported the imaging findings. They marked the PMCT feature of the presence of foam-covered airway fluid or high-attenuation deposit in the airways of cadavers. Also the fluid presence was noticed in the para-nasal cavity, mastoid air cell fluid, gastric distends and contents, proving the facts of death due to drowning [9] in 2010 reported the applicability of PMCT in determination of cause of death in case of a middle aged male who died after falling in a sewage pool. PMCT imaging showed the presence of blood accumulation in the right external auditory canal, right humerus fracture, subarachnoid space possessing small hemorrhages, left temporal lobe showing brain contusion injuries, the occipital scalp showed occurrence of scratch and bruise injuries on the right side. All these injuries in combination may have cause unconscious leading to coma, thus making the individual unable to rescue himself from pool. Other findings such as presence of fluid in the air passage, paranasal sinuses, gastric and duodenal expansion also indicates that the victim was continuously breathing and swallowing even after falling into the water. Further the proof that water has entered into the respiratory and circulatory systems was established from the PMCT findings showing opacity in both the lungs (**Figure 1**) [10]. Jian et al. performed a study involving drowned rabbit model. They compared these animal models of hemorrhagic shock and mechanical asphyxia. The CT values indicated that the lungs volumes were significantly higher ($P < 0.05$) thus signifying that the virtopsy characteristics can reflect the important features in case of antemortem drowning [9, 11].

In cases of firearms injury, the determination of permanent damage caused by the bullet, entry & exit of bullet, diversion of bullet by anatomical structure can be studied in detailed by the use of Multislice spiral CT. Gibb [12] demonstrated the use of CT in real cases and animal models and identified the several characteristics of injuries caused by different types of firearms and ammunition (**Figure 2**). Harcke et al. [13] utilized CT scans of less intensity for 3D projection and 3D volume reconstruction on the complete body of cadavers possessing gunshot injuries. They

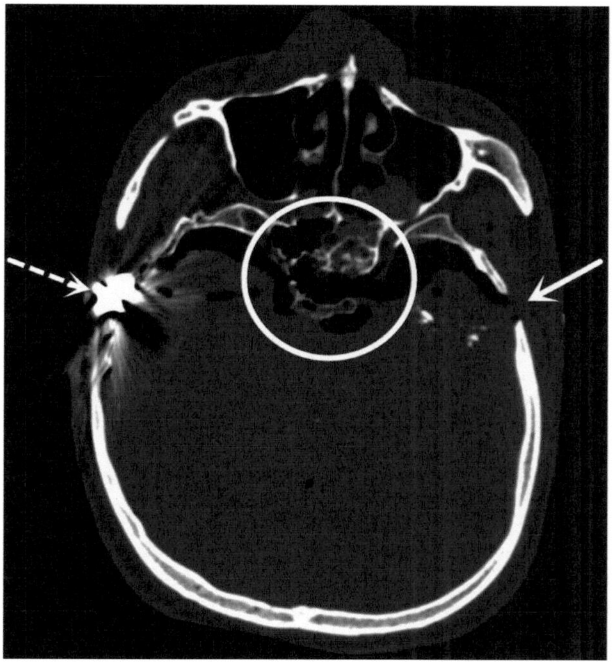

Figure 1.
PMCT revealed the bullet's entrance (white arrow), the skull fracture caused by the bullet (white circle), and the bullet and the exit (dotted arrow).

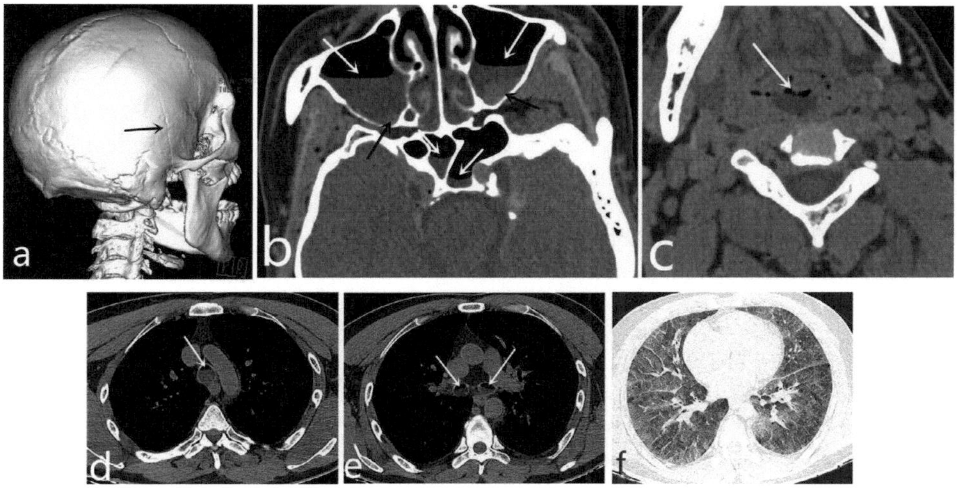

Figure 2.
(a) SSD reconstruct revealed the fracture of right temporal bone (black arrow). (b) Fluid in the paranasal sinuses (white arrows), and dense sediment (black arrows). (c) Fluid in the throat (white arrow). (d) and (e) Fluid in the trachea (white arrows). (f) The diffuse ground-glass opacities in both lungs.

examined the bone damaged, projectile trajectory as well as bone fragments in the body. The technology proved to be very significant at the level of identifying the perforation and penetration caused by firearms. Further, Karger et al. [14] studied tissue

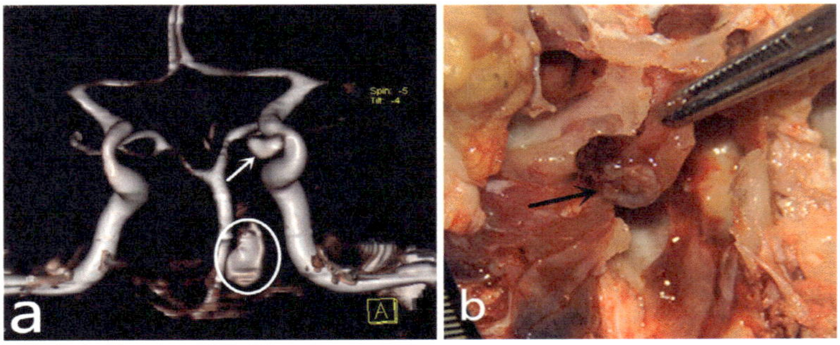

Figure 3.
(a) PMCTA results showed a leakage of the contrast agent from the C3 segment of the left internal carotid artery (white arrow) into the adjacent left sphenoidsinus (white circle), suggesting an aneurysm. (b)An aneurysm inside the left sphenoid sinus (black arrow) was confirmed by autopsy, consistent to the PMCTA results.

disruption in case of gunshot to the head by using MRI and PMCT. They observed that the permanent tract of tissue damage was very well defined as well as the fragments of the bone were easily located inside, which could not have been identified in case of normal traditional autopsy. In china, a police officer committed suicide due to depression whose PMCT was performed. The data clearly inferred the bullet entrance & exit hole, skull fracture, trajectory of bullet and other injuries along with the manner of death decipherment as shown in **Figure 3**.

Virtopsy technology has shown its wide application in the field of forensic odontology. Human identification and age estimation can be achieved via dentition structure as it comprehends multiple teeth identifiers [15]. Dental identification encompasses the comparison between ante-mortem and post mortem evidence, analysis of dentition profiles of PM victim and dental DNA examination [16]. In certain cases the access to the dentition or oral cavity postmortem data is hindered (e.g. rigor mortis condition) the use of virtopsy can prove to be accurate and rapid way to shelter the information [17]. Oesterhelweg et al. [18] described a case where a foreign material (food bolus) got struck in respiratory tract. In case of traditional autopsy the depth of these material would not have been determined but the use of CT and MRI overcome these facts. Personal identification was achieved by superimposition and comparing the data of ante mortem orthopantomo grams and postmortem reconstructed panoramic imaging of cranial CT scans [19, 20]. Dentistry helps in the age estimation in case of charred bodies where the use of CT scans have proven its application in a well-defined manner as described by Dedouit et al. [21]. Personal identification was also achieved in cases of the Australian bushfire victims through the CT scans based on age estimation techniques [22–24]. Researchers have demonstrated the use of Virtual Autopsy in case of fire mass disaster by simulating the complete scenario. Jackowski et al. [25] utilized different restoration materials namely composites, ceramics and temporary fillings under high temperature and the CT scans of the same were studied [26].

Death occurring due to cerebral hemorrhage are observed very frequently in forensic investigation. In 2017, Qian et al. [27] studied a case where the individual died due to rupture of cerebrovascular distortion. The PMCT scan of brain's right frontal region indicated massive hemorrhage ranging up to the ventricular system. Histological examination also established the facts of PMCT angiography that the death was caused by an arteriovenous distortion (**Figure 4**).

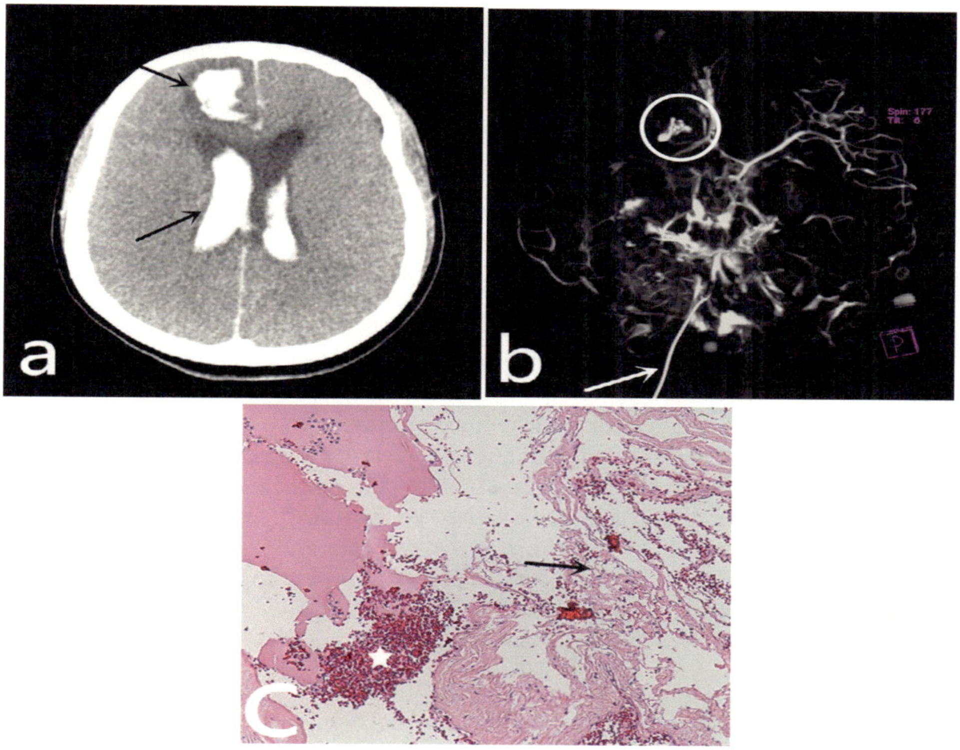

Figure 4.
(a) Massive hemorrhage in the brain's right frontal region, extending into the ventricular system (white arrow); (b)a mass of irregular, tortuous vessels in areas of hemorrhage in the right frontal lobe of the brain (white circle); a contrast agent was injected into the basilar artery (white arrow); (c) Lumps of abnormal blood vessels within the region of hematoma (star); small blood vessels were dilated and tortuous, and the thickness of the vessel wall varied (black arrow).

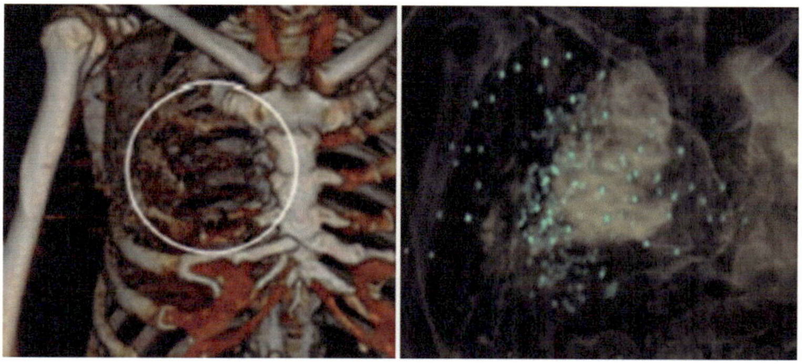

Figure 5.
Left: computed tomography three-dimensional reconstruction shows fractures in right ribs 2–4 (white circles); Right: computed tomography three-dimensional reconstruction shows scattered bullets (blue-green).

In 2017, Shao et al. [28] executed PMCT angiography on a deceased who suffered a head injury during a traffic accident. The deceases had fractures of frontal and sphenoid bones-left. The PMCT angiography showed rupturing of internal carotid artery aneurysm. Consequently, the location of the injury spotted by the virtopsy, autopsy and histo-pathological examination confirmed that the sinusoidal vascular injury was a pseudo aneurysm initiated because of the traffic accident. The application of virtopsy can prove to be applicable in cases where the real cause of the damage in not known by the investigator (**Figure 5**).

3. Reconstruction

Michael J. Thali et al., [29] established the use of 3D data centered on geometric methodology. It involves the use of radiological CT/MRI, scanning photogrammetry, and optical surface which examine the topography and internal injuries in case of living as well as dead bodies in non-invasive and non-destructive manner. These results can prove too significant for the reconstruction in crime scene cases. The use of the data fusing and animation techniques various reconstructive questions can be answered with respect to the patterned injuries and their link with the suspect or injury causing instrument. The documentation in forensic aspects was limited to the traditional 2D photography, radiographs, sketches and witness description. This recent development in 3D imaging has described a new approach in the forensic examination and reconstruction. Michael J. Thali et al. applied these technology in automobile accident reconstruction cases. They created 3D data of the injuries and

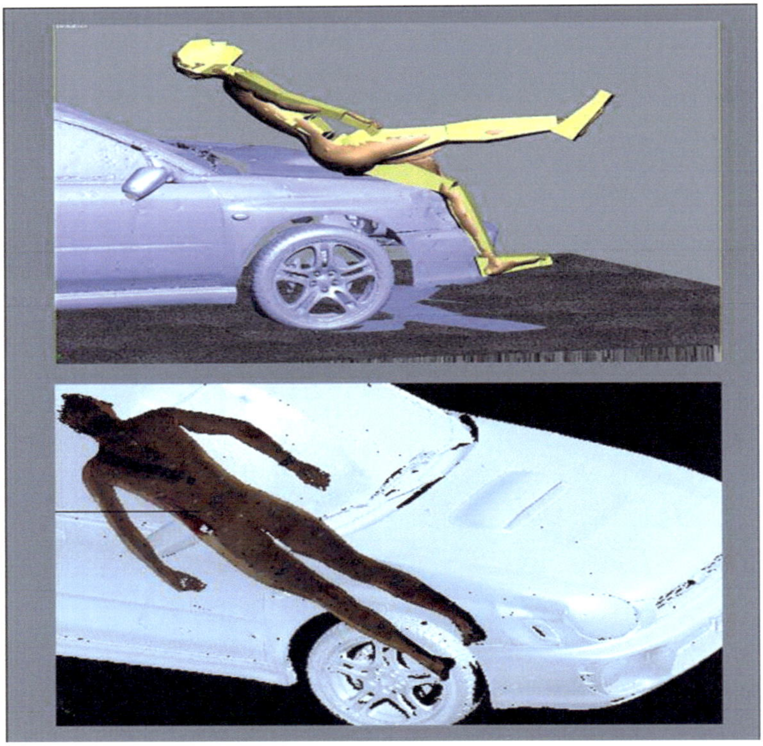

Figure 6.
3D geometric data for forensic analysis and reconstructive animation are possible. Investigative opinions can be analyzed, helping to develop an expert opinion.

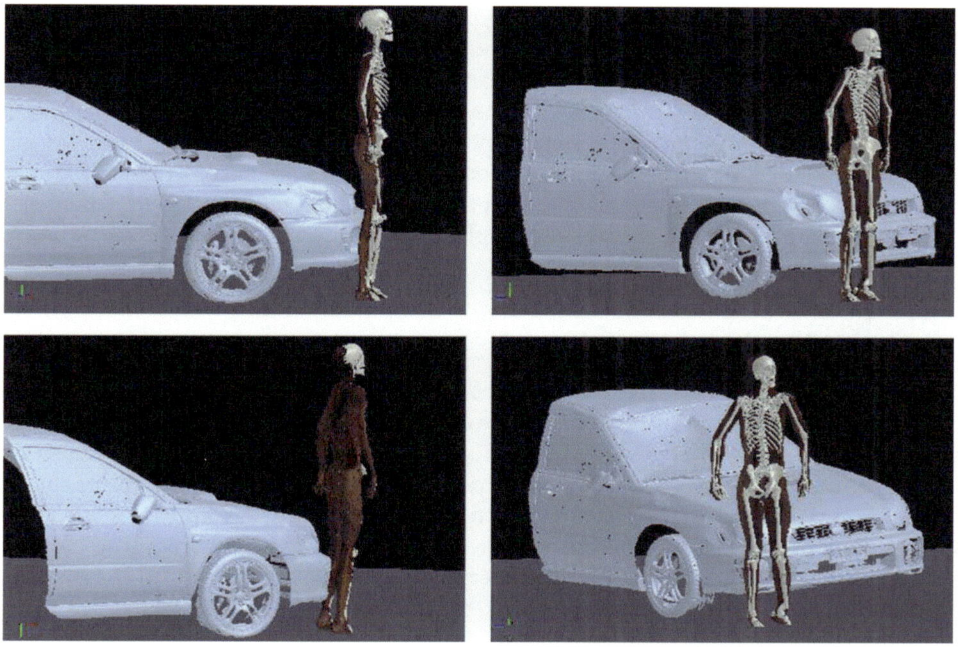

Figure 7.
Implementation of the skeletal and joint information into the data set of the car allows for individual and correct (real data based) simulation of movements of the body.

link it to the animation created data with respect to the body injuries and vehicular damage. The detailed measurements and analysis of the damages caused to the vehicle not only allowed to determine the impact points but also helped in force determination and vehicle speed. 3D real data documentation opens up a new horizon in the examination of forensic evidences, reconstruction and thus creating an animation of the incidences pertaining to case investigation as shown in **Figures 6** and 7. In 2007, Buck et al. [30] generated the 3D models of human injuries and vehicles during the traffic accident by the application of high-resolution surface scanning and multi slice CT/MRI scanning. The scanning provided information useful in judging the positions of vehicles. Various authors showed the use of 3D scanning in vehicular accidents with respect to the injuries examination, cause of death and vehicle damage. They concluded that a combination of PMCT and autopsy can prove to be the best way for the determination of cause and manner of the death in traffic accidents [31–35].

4. Advantages

The most important advantage of the technique is it is non-destructive method of examination which is scalpel free mode. It is an ethical fruition of the technology which make the body examination more acceptable without hurting the sentiments of the family as well as maintains the body architecture. It is less time consuming and the data generated in a manner of images is easily transferable, can be reused for future studies also. It proves to be most effective way of examination of injuries and establishing the relationship with the probable weapon used for the commission of crime. The 3D scanning also adds in the weightage of the forensic report and make the work easy for the experts in describing the reconstructions or animations of the case investigations. The examination can be performed with ease without causing any damage to the authenticity in a non-destructive manner in both living and non-living individuals. Forensic documentation can be done via storing the data in images format obtained from photogrammetric and 3D optical scanning. Virtual autopsy also reduces the chances of the infections, radionuclide, toxic substances or other bio-hazards. The imaging system has come out to be a steadfast tool in modern forensic examination with various aspects of its application in different fields.

5. Disadvantages

Although the technique has wide advantages but does possess certain flaws into it. Certain pathological conditions such as the level of infection into the cadaver, changes in physical features namely color, spoor and small tissue damages cannot be defined or may get miss. The system does not have database which can prove useful for the comparison purpose. It becomes difficult to differentiate between ante-mortem and post mortem injuries. Accuracy can become questionable if the data merging happens from multiple technology also can create a complete dependency on the imagery system.

Conflict of interest

The authors declare no conflict of interest.

Author details

Pooja Ahuja* and Niha Ansari
National Forensic Sciences University, Gandhinagar, India

*Address all correspondence to: pooja.ahuja@nfsu.ac.in

References

[1] Franco A, Souza P, Coudyzer W, Thevissen P, Jacobs R, Willems G. Virtual autopsy in forensic sciences and its application in the forensic odontology. Revista Odonto Ciência. 2012;**27**:5-9. DOI: 10.1590/S1980-65232012000100001.

[2] Pomara C, Fineschi V, Scalzo G, Guglielmi G. Virtopsy versus digital autopsy: virtuous autopsy. La Radiologia Medica. 2009;**114**:1367-1382

[3] Rosário Junior AF, Couto Souza PH, Coudyzer W, Thevissen P, Willems G, Jacobs R. Virtual autopsy in forensic sciences and its application in the forensic odontology. Revista Odonto Ciência. 2012;**27**(1):5-9

[4] Biswas UK, Hossain MA, Moinuddin KM, Khan NT. Virtopsy: New dimension in the field of forensic medicine communities. Journal of ZH Sikder Women's Medical College. 2021;**3**(1):30-33

[5] The future is Virtopsy: Sequence format (NeueZuricherZeitung) Telecast [Internet]. 2006. Available from: www.Virtopsy.com/index.php?id=45

[6] Surabhi MT, Bhateja S, Arora G. Virtopsy: An aid in forensic investigation. IP International Journal of Forensic Medicine and Toxicological Sciences. 2019;**4**(4):95-98

[7] Gupta S, Gupta R, Singh VS, Dhingra V. Virtopsy: A new innovation for forensic science. Journal of Forensic Chemistry and Toxicology. 2015;**1**(1):43-46

[8] Levy AD, Harcke HT, Getz JM, Mallak CT, Caruso JL, Pearse L, et al. Virtual autopsy: Two and three dimensional multidetection CT findings in drowning with autopsy comparison. Radiology. 2007;**243**:862-868

[9] Yucong W, Haibiao Z, Ran L, Haidong Z, Dong Z, Xu W, et al. Application of virtopsy in forensic pathology. Journal of Forensic Science and Medicine. 2021;**7**:14-23

[10] Wan L, Song YX, Li ZD, Liu NG, Wang YH, Wang MW, et al. The approach of virtual autopsy (VIRTOPSY) by postmortem multi-slice computed tomography (PMCT) in China for forensic pathology. Forensic Imaging. 2020;**20**:200361

[11] Jian J, Deng D, Wan L, Zou DH, Wang ZQ, Liu NG, et al. Characteristic changes and 3D virtual measurement of lung CT image parameters in the drowning rabbit model. Journal of Forensic Medicine. 2019;**35**:1-4

[12] Gibb IE. Computed tomography of projectile injuries. Clinical Radiology. 2008;**63**:1168

[13] Harcke HT, Levy AD, Getz JM, Robinson SR. MDCT analysis of projectile injury in forensic investigation. AJR. American Journal of Roentgenology. 2008;**190**(2):106-111

[14] Karger B, Puskas Z, Ruwald B, Teige K, Schuirer G. Morphological findings in the brain after experimental gunshots using radiology, pathology and histology. International Journal of Legal Medicine. 1998;**111**(6):314-319

[15] Thali MJ, Jackowski C, Oesterhelweg L, Ross S, Dirnhofer R. Virtopsy – The swiss virtual autopsy approach. Legal Medicine. 2007;**9**:100-104

[16] Girish KL, Rahman FS, Tippu SR. Dental DNA fingerprinting in identification of human remains. Journal of Forensic Dental Sciences. 2010;**2**:63-68

[17] Jackowski C, Wyss M, Persson A, Classens M, Thali MJ, Lussi A. Ultra-high-resolution dual-source CT for forensic dental visualization – Discrimination of ceramic and composite fillings. International Journal of Legal Medicine. 2008;**122**:301-307

[18] Oesterhelweg L, Bolliger SA, Thali MJ, Ross S. Postmortem imaging of laryngeal foreign bodies. Archives of Pathology & Laboratory Medicine. 2010;**133**:806-810

[19] Dirnhofer R, Jackowski C, Vock P, Potter K, Thali MJ. Virtopsy – Minimally invasive, imaging guided virtual autopsy. Radio Graphics. 2006;**26**:1305-1333

[20] Birngruber CG, Obert M, Ramsthaler F, Kreutz K, Verhoff MA. Comparative dental radiographic identification using flat panel CT. Forensic Science International. 2011;**209**:31-34

[21] Dedouit F, Telmon N, Costaglioga R, Otal P, Joffre F, Rougé D. Virtual anthropology and forensic identification: Report of one case. Forensic Science International. 2007;**173**:182-187

[22] Bassed RB, Hill AJ. The use of computed tomography (CT) to estimate age in the 2009 Victorian bushfire victims: A case report. Forensic Science International. 2011;**205**:48-51

[23] O'donell C, Lino M, Mansharan K, Leditscke J, Woodford N. Contribution of post mortem multidetector CT scanning to the identification of the deceased in a mass disaster: Experience gained from the 2009 Victorian bushfires. Forensic Science International. 2011;**205**:15-28

[24] Cordner SM, Woodford N, Bassed R. Forensic aspects of the 2009 Victorian bushfires disaster. Forensic Science International. 2011;**205**:2-7

[25] Kawasumi Y, Kawabata T, Sugai Y, Usui A, Hosokai Y, Sato M, et al. Assessment of the relationship between drowning and fluid accumulation in the paranasal sinuses on post-mortem computed tomography. European Journal of Radiology. 2012;**81**(12):3953-3955

[26] Zou D, Shao Y, Zhang J, Wan L, Qin Z, Liu N, et al. Determination of a Newborn with lethal type H osteogenesis imperfect and other anomalies using autopsy and postmortem MSCT: A case report. Journal of Forensic Medicine. 2016;**1**:69-73

[27] Qian H, Shao Y, Li Z, Huang P, Zou D, Liu N, et al. Diagnosis of a cerebral arteriovenous malformation using isolated brain computed tomography angiography: Case report. The American Journal of Forensic Medicine and Pathology. 2016;**37**(3):201-204

[28] Shao Y, Wan L, Zhang J, Li Z, Liu N, Huang P, et al. Post-mortem computed tomography angiography using left ventricle cardiac puncture: A whole-body, angiographic approach. PLoS One. 2017;**12**(8):1-7

[29] Thali MJ, Braun M, Buck U, Aghayev E, Jackowski C, Vock P, et al. VIRTOPSY—Scientific documentation, reconstruction and animation in forensic: Individual and real 3D data based geo-metric approach including optical body/object surface and radiological CT/MRI scanning. Journal of Forensic Sciences. 2005;**50**(2):428-442

[30] Thali MJ, Braun M, Dirnhofer R. Optical 3D surface digitizing in forensic medicine: 3D documentation of skin and bone injuries. Forensic Science International. 2003;**137**(2-3):203-208

[31] Oliver WR, Chancellor AS, Soltys M, Symon J, Cullip T, Rosenman J, et al. Three-dimensional reconstruction of

a bullet path: Validation by computed radiography. Journal of Forensic Sciences. 1995;**40**(2):321-324

[32] Subke J, Wehner HD, Wehner F, Szczepaniak S. Streifenlichttopometrie (SLT): A new method for the three-dimensional photorealistic forensic documentation in colour. Forensic Science International. 2000;**113**(1-3):289-295

[33] Thali M, Vock P. Role of and techniques in forensic imaging. In: Payen-James J, Busuttil A, Smock W, editors. Forensic Medicine: Clinical and Pathological Aspects. London: Greenwich Medical Media; 2003. pp. 731-745

[34] Thali MJ, Braun M, Brueschweiler W, Dirnhofer R. 'Morphological imprint': Determination of the injury-causing weapon from the wound morphology using forensic 3D/CAD-supported photogrammetry. Forensic Science International. 2003;**132**(3):177-181

[35] Thali MJ, Braun M, Bruschweiler W, Dirnhofer R. Matching tire tracks on the head using forensic photogrammetry. Forensic Science International. 2000;**113**(1-3):281-287